THE ATLAS OF
DISEASE

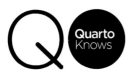

First published in 2018 by White Lion Publishing,
an imprint of The Quarto Group.
The Old Brewery, 6 Blundell Street,
London, N7 9BH,
United Kingdom
T (0)20 7700 6700
www.QuartoKnows.com

A catalogue record for this book is available from the British Library.

ISBN 978 1 78131 790 7
Ebook ISBN 978 1 78131 880 5

10 9 8 7 6 5 4 3 2 1

Medical history consultant: Dr Dora Vargha, Lecturer in Medical Humanities, University of Exeter
Design by Paileen Currie and Ginny Zeal
Map Illustrations by Lovell Johns

Printed in Malaysia

THE ATLAS OF
DISEASE

Mapping deadly epidemics and contagion
from the plague to the zika virus

SANDRA HEMPEL

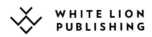
WHITE LION
PUBLISHING

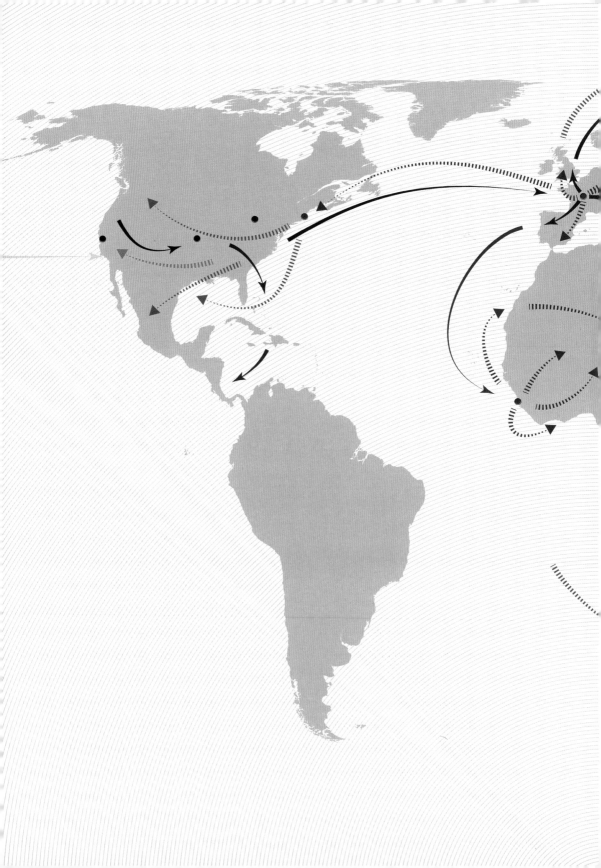

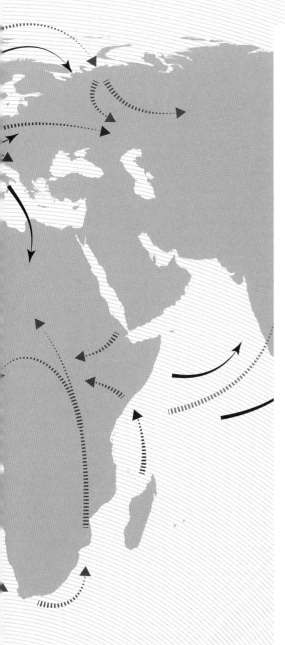

Contents

Introduction

||||||||||||||||||

The story of how deadly diseases invaded our world makes fascinating reading. From the moment that scourges such as plague, smallpox and syphilis first struck at human populations, the unfolding narrative would encompass so much more than medicine and science. For in tracking the paths of epidemics over the centuries, we can draw clear parallels with the story of our own progress, from when we first began living together in settlements and herding animals, through the growing interaction between different nations and civilisations, to the mass movements of people in the name of trade, exploration and conquest.

And we also see the terrible consequences of epidemics at particular times and in particular places, not only in terms of individual suffering, but also in their social and economic effects, particularly on some of the most deprived groups of people.

Since the mid-nineteenth century, maps have played a vital role in helping us to unravel the mysteries of how diseases spread. The experts have used them to work out how best to prevent, or at least to contain, future outbreaks. One of the first and best-known examples of disease mapping was the work of the physician Dr John Snow during a virulent outbreak of cholera in London's Soho in 1854. Around 600 people died, 200 of them during the course of one night.

At that time no one understood how cholera was transmitted, which meant that doctors could not begin to fathom how to stop it. No other disease behaved like cholera, and the medical profession had been baffled for centuries by the way that it struck apparently at random and killed hundreds or even thousands of people within days. Cholera is the human species' fastest killer disease and in the 1800s millions died in a series of cholera pandemics that swept the globe.

Snow was convinced that cholera was being spread through contaminated drink-

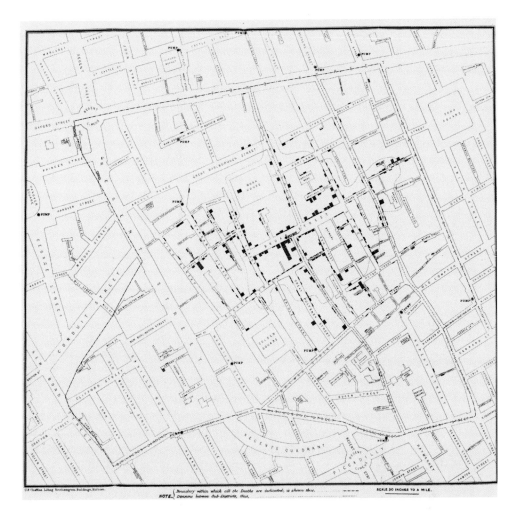

Above John Snow's iconic map of the 1854 cholera epidemic around Broad Street, Soho.

ing water, which would explain all of its seeming inconsistencies, but this idea was then too revolutionary for the medical establishment to take seriously. After the Soho epidemic, in an effort to prove his theory, Snow took to the streets, knocking on doors, asking how many people had died in each house. He then plotted his data onto a street plan and that now iconic map revealed that the vast majority of deaths were clustered around the pump well in Broad Street: at every point where

it was more convenient to go to another pump, the fatalities tailed off.

For his work in Soho and also for a similar, larger piece of research in south London, John Snow is known as the father of epidemiology, the branch of medical science that studies the incidence, distribution and determinants of disease. Epidemiologists are interested not in individual patients but in the wider, public health picture. Put simply, they look at who gets sick and why, and because they investigate sudden outbreaks of disease, they are known as the medical detectives.

In this atlas, we use statistics to plot the course of some of the pivotal and devastating epidemics and pandemics caused by the most virulent diseases across the centuries. The information is presented in a series of specially commissioned maps that bring the dry data to life in a way that lists and tables never can. Some of the maps, like the spread of the 1918 Spanish flu epidemic (see pages 26–7), illustrate huge historic pandemics, while others focus on more localised outbreaks, confined to a particular town or small region, such as the spread of measles in Fiji from the HMS *Dido* in 1875 (see page 48). And alongside them are historical maps and illustrations showing how different diseases were viewed at different times in history and also how, through the ages, the authorities tried to instruct the public about how to protect themselves.

The accompanying commentaries explain the background to the routes on the maps – the wars, the explorations and exploitations, the panics and the victim-blaming. The text also examines the medical and social contexts, in particular how doctors struggled to understand how and why people were falling sick and the attempts of different societies to make sense of the disaster that appeared to have hit them from out of the blue. In fact, the word epidemiology comes from the Greek, 'epi' meaning 'upon' and 'demos', 'the people' – so an epidemic is something that falls upon the masses.

There are some striking stories. There is the blame game that broke out at the end of the fifteenth century when syphilis first struck in Europe, with each nation holding another responsible for the disease. There are the heart-breaking seventeenth-century reports of the slave ships arriving in the Caribbean with their human 'cargoes' decimated by dysentery. There are the prisoners in Newgate jail in the eighteenth century who agreed to be inoculated against smallpox in return for escaping the gallows. And there is the heroism of the young American doctor in the early twentieth century who acted as a guinea pig in the fight to control yellow fever and died in the attempt.

But this is not only the story of the great plagues of the past. Today, despite the extraordinary advances in microbiology and medicine of the twentieth and twenty-first centuries, the human race is still engaged in a hard-fought struggle against the deadly pathogens that, despite all the weapons now in our armoury, all too often seem to be one jump ahead.

In the 1970s, a young student considering a career in research into infectious diseases was advised against it. There was no point, his professor told him. Infectious diseases were now all but conquered: there was nothing left to do.

Sadly, the professor turned out to be horribly wrong but at the time his was a perfectly reasonable view. Thanks to vaccination and antibiotics, the killer diseases that had rampaged across the world for centuries, terrorising and ravaging entire populations, seemed finally to be on the retreat. In 1979, smallpox was officially declared eradicated from the globe and many people believed that the others were surely set soon to follow.

Forty years later though smallpox remains the only human disease to gain this distinction. And while others are tantalisingly close to being conquered, they have proved extraordinarily persistent, with some even staging something of a come back. Then there are the new diseases that emerge without warning and are able to traverse the globe in hours, thanks to international travel. Even more worrying is the growing resistance to antibiotics, by far the most effective treatment that we have ever possessed.

In 2002, a previously unknown type of pneumonia appeared in China. Severe acute respiratory syndrome, or SARS, went on to kill over 700 people across North and South America, Europe and Asia. This new pathogen turned out to be related to the common cold, which has been with us for centuries as nothing more than a mild irritant.

Ebola was first identified in 1976 but the condition had attracted little attention, confined as it was to small outbreaks in Central Africa. Then in 2014, it suddenly burst its bounds, striking first in West Africa where it had previously been unknown, and then appearing in different parts of the world, including Europe and the United States.

Fortunately for the cause of public health, the student, Peter Piot, ignored his mentor's advice and spent his career studying infectious diseases. Unfortunately though for the human race, over the following more than 40 years, infectious diseases proved to be extremely fertile ground for researchers. Piot went on to become one of the world's foremost clinical microbiologists, the first person to identify the ebola virus and a leading figure in unravelling the mysteries of another deadly new infection, the human immunodeficiency virus, or HIV.

By 2016, the HIV and AIDS pandemic had been responsible for at least 35 million deaths, and many millions more people were known to be carrying the virus, the majority of them without access to life-saving drugs. For anything on a comparable scale, it is necessary to go back to the fourteenth century and the Black Death, which killed an estimated 60 per cent of Europe's eighty million population and and between seventy-five million to two hundred million across the world.

In the fourteenth century, with no knowledge of microbiology and with religion playing a central role in people's lives, the Black Death was seen as possibly a punishment from God, as other diseases such as leprosy had long been seen. But while we like to think of ourselves as more enlightened and educated than our ancient and medieval ancestors, the victims of HIV and AIDS were also ostracised, and some people claimed that the disease was divine retribution for a dissolute lifestyle. In the same way, people with leprosy, or Hansen's disease as it is now known, still face discrimination in some parts of the world.

Behind each of these maps then there is fear and suffering, but there is also the relentless quest for knowledge that would allow the human race to fight back against deadly enemies that are still proving remarkably resourceful.

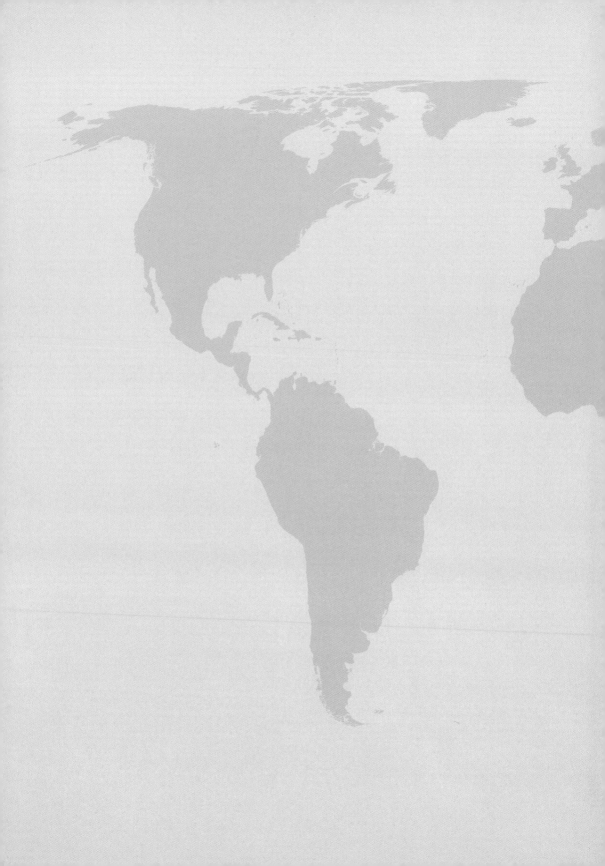

SECTION 1
AIRBORNE

||||||||||||||||||||||||||||||||||||||||||||

Diphtheria

|||||||||||||||||||||

Causal agent	Bacterium *Corynebacterium diphtheriae*
Transmission	Respiratory route and direct contact
Symptoms	Weakness, sore throat, fever, swollen neck glands, thick grey coating in the throat or nose
Incidence and deaths	Around 5,000 cases a year worldwide. Fatal in 5–10 per cent of cases.
Prevalence	Endemic in many countries in Asia, the South Pacific, the Middle East, Eastern Europe and in Haiti and the Dominican Republic. Rare in industrialised countries.
Prevention	Vaccination
Treatment	Antitoxins and antibiotics
Global strategy	Childhood vaccination programmes but the World Health Organization (WHO) describes diphtheria as a 'forgotten' disease

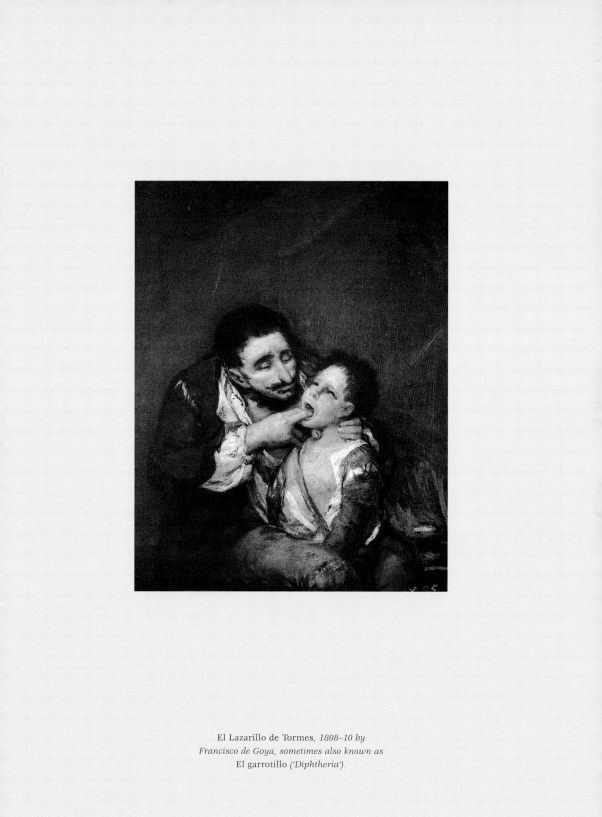

El Lazarillo de Tormes, *1808–10 by*
Francisco de Goya, sometimes also known as
El garrotillo *('Diphtheria')*.

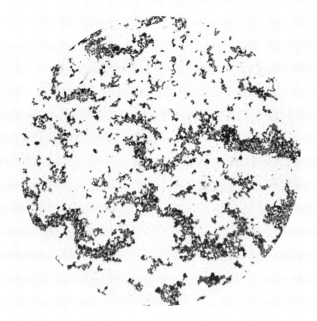

Above: *Microscopic image of diphtheria bacteria,*
Corynebacterium diphtheriae.

In 1859, *The Lancet* published a report on the sudden appearance of 'a strange type of disease'. The author, a surgeon at the West London Hospital called Ernest Hart, described the unknown sickness as 'distressing in its symptoms, rapid in its progress, intractable, and communicable by infection and by contagion'. It also 'acted with severity in confined areas of population' and left 'terrible traces of its passage', he wrote.

Hart said it was important to find out if this malady was entirely new to the world or had, in fact, re-emerged from foreign lands and previous centuries. One thing, however, was clear: 'The most experienced surgeons ... find themselves called upon to combat an unknown enemy, and one whose mode of attack is new to them.'

The return of an old disease

While diphtheria's origins and its route into Europe are unknown, it was not new to Britain in the 1850s. Various medical reports in previous centuries describe what appear to be its symptoms, and in 1821 the French physician Pierre Bretonneau had identified diphtheria as a separate disease from other childhood illnesses.

The German scientist Friedrich Loeffler – who identified the bacterium *Corynebacterium diphtheriae* as being responsible for the disease in 1884 – claimed there were no descriptions of diphtheria in the writings of any of the great classical Greek physicians. But others believe that Hippocrates, the 'father of Western medicine', referred to it in the fifth century BC. Regardless, many experts, including Loeffler, accept that the infection was well-known in ancient Egypt, Syria and Palestine.

Some of the more recent accounts in the West of a disease that appears to be diphtheria date from sixth-century France, from Rome in 856 and 1004, and from parts of the Byzantine empire in 1039. Loeffler also refers to what he believed was an outbreak in England in 1389, which he said killed many children. As with scarlet fever – with which it was often confused – diphtheria favours the young.

The Strangler

The first recorded major epidemic seems to have been in France in 1562–98 during the religious wars between the Catholics and the Huguenots. It reached Paris in 1576. It was followed by an infamous epidemic in Spain in 1583–1618, where it was dubbed *El garrotillo* – 'The Strangler' – and the year of 1613 was referred to as *Ano de los garrotillos*, the 'Year of the Strangler'.

Diphtheria was known as 'the Strangler' because of its unpleasant tendency to suffocate its victim. The bacterium destroys the lining of the throat, causing dead tissue and pus to merge together over the site, forming a tough leathery membrane known as a pseudomembrane. Any attempt to remove it rips at the live tissue beneath, causing massive bleeding. If it is left in place, however, the membrane blocks the patient's airway. Even if the sufferer manages to survive the effects of the membrane, the toxin can invade the body, damaging organs and nerves.

Something in the air?

In the great medical science breakthroughs of the second half of the nineteenth century, doctors were beginning to understand the role germs played in spreading epidemic disease. In the late 1800s and early 1900s, bacteriologists like Loeffler were fast identifying the different pathogens responsible for different diseases and the infections' various means of transmission.

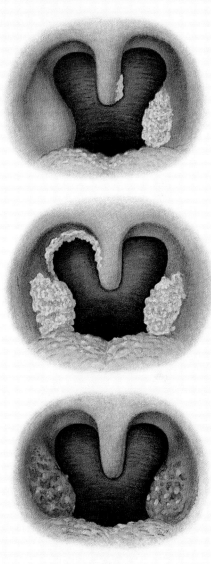

Above: *The symptoms of diphtheria, as seen affecting the mouth.*

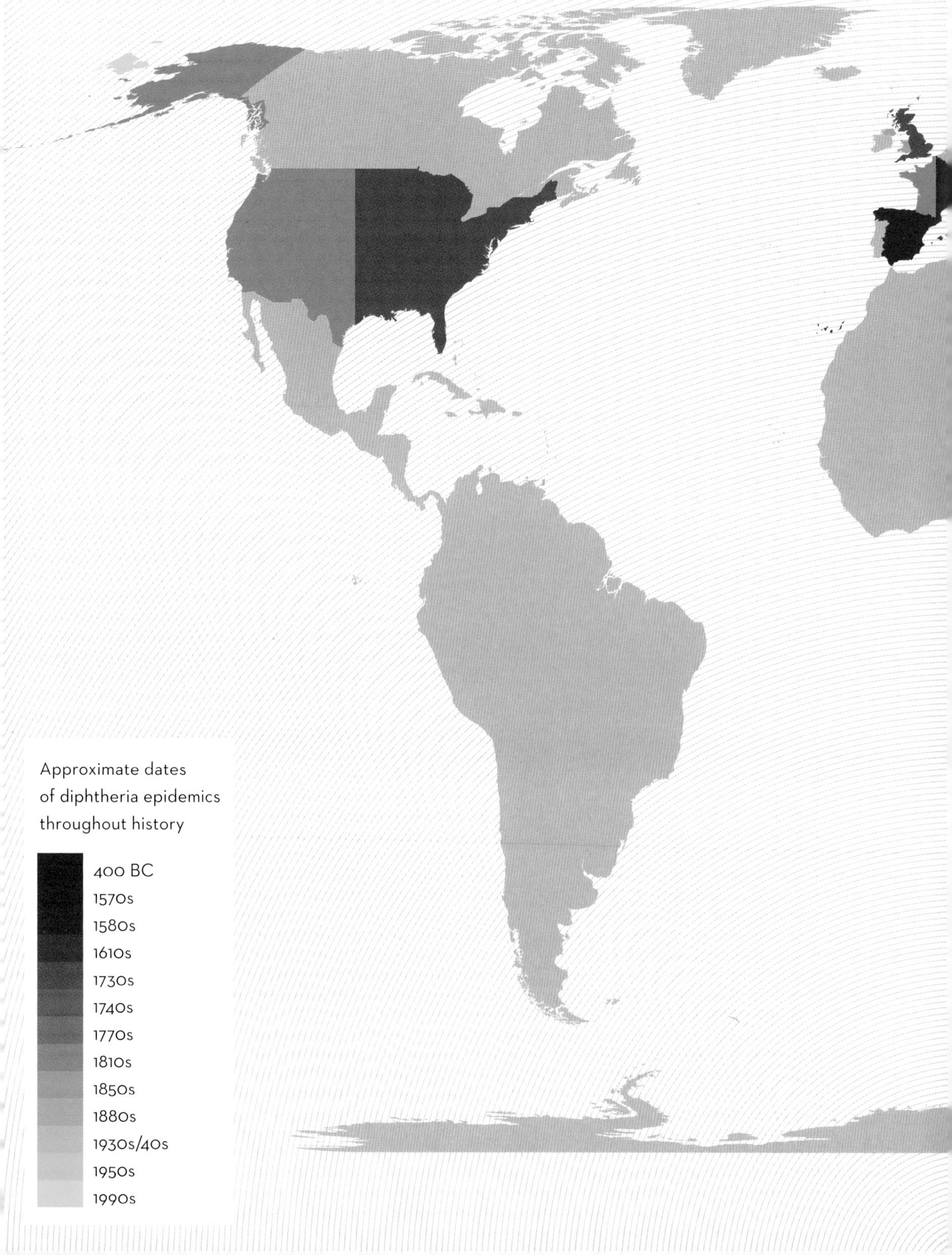

Approximate dates
of diphtheria epidemics
throughout history

400 BC
1570s
1580s
1610s
1730s
1740s
1770s
1810s
1850s
1880s
1930s/40s
1950s
1990s

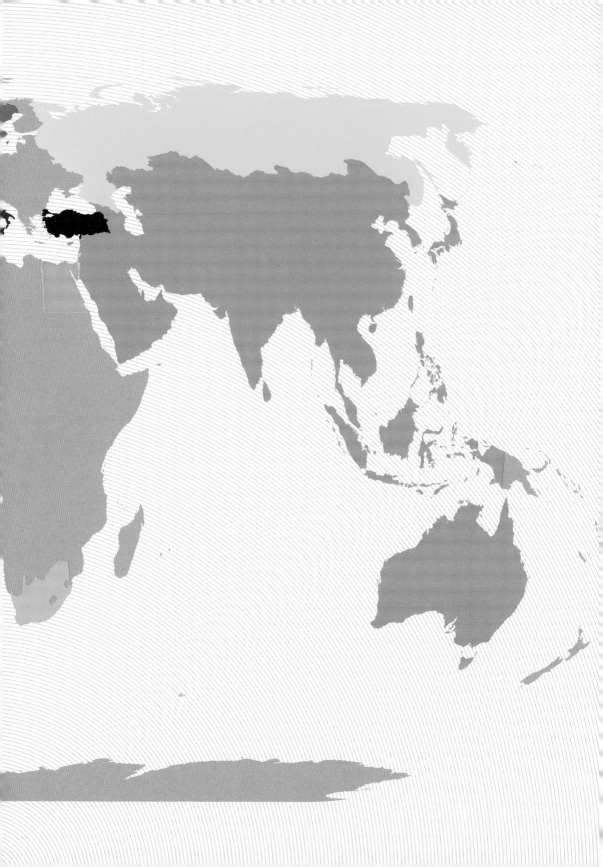

Diphtheria, which is highly infectious, is mainly caught by inhaling droplets released into the air by an infected person's coughs or sneezes. It can also be passed on through direct contact with bacteria, for example, in mucous or on surfaces and objects.

Back in the 1850s, however, when the mystery epidemic hit Britain, the centuries-old theory of miasmatism still held sway. Foul smells, or miasma, from decaying organic matter – bad food, rotting carcasses and excreta, for example – or emanating from marshlands and stagnant water, were thought to contain the 'poisons' that caused disease. Other factors such as the climate determined which particular disease prevailed.

This may explain why in 1859 Ernest Hart looked to the weather and the environment for clues. He could find none and waxed lyrical in his bafflement. The disease 'has swept across the marshy lowlands of Essex and the bleak moors of Yorkshire', he noted. Of other parts of the country, he wrote:

> It has traversed the flowery lanes of Devon and the wild flats of Cornwall that are swept by the sea-breeze. It has seated itself on the banks of the Thames, scaled the romantic heights of North Wales and descended into the Cornish mines. Commencing in the spring months, it has continued through the summer, and if extremes of temperature have appeared to lend it fresh vigour and the heat of the dog-days, or the severe frosts and sleet of winter have fostered its strength, yet moderate temperature has not greatly abated its influence, and it has struck a blow here and there through all the seasons.

As late as 1908 the medical officer for Croydon in south London still thought it worth inspecting all 310 houses where the disease had struck on his patch, to see if there was a link between diphtheria and defective drains. As he already suspected, however, no such connection could be found.

An escalation of deaths

Until the nineteenth century, the disease commonly struck in tightly contained outbreaks; for example, in a hamlet, a school or a family. It might cause terrible losses within those small confines but tended not to spread further.

All this changed in Britain during the nineteenth-century Industrial Revolution when people flocked into the towns in search of work and were crowded into slum housing. The pattern of disease was still localised outbreaks within communities or districts, but those outbreaks were now numerous, more widely spread and affected many districts at the same time. In the late nineteenth and early twentieth centuries, diphtheria turned from an occasional tragedy into a major killer. The explosion of disease led to claims it had been imported from overseas and for a while it was known as 'Boulogne sore throat'.

But as well as the change in living conditions, a more virulent strain of the bacterium may well have been involved: between 30 and 50 per cent of children who caught diphtheria in the nineteenth century died from it. In 1885 the medical officer for the parish of Hanover Square in central London reported: 'Diphtheria caused no less than 35 deaths, being the largest number recorded in the parish in any year, and nearly 2½ times the annual average for the preceding 10 years; being also an increase of 10 on the number for

1884.' Diphtheria had been 'exceedingly prevalent' throughout London since 1883.

In the following year, the medical officer for St Mary Abbott's in Kensington reported thirty deaths from diphtheria, more than for any year for a decade. He couldn't account for the increase but wondered if it might be due to better diagnosis rather than a real increase. Both factors probably had a part to play.

New breakthroughs

From the late nineteenth century and into the twentieth century, great progress was made both in the treatment and prevention of diphtheria. The first advance was the development of what is known as an antitoxin that harnesses the body's own attempts to neutralise the bacterium's poison. This made the disease much less lethal and in many cases curable. There was also another important benefit: the need to mass-produce antitoxins played a strong part in integrating pharmaceutical production with research.

Then in 1923, in France, came a vaccine. An epidemic in the United States in 1921–5 killed around 15,500 people, with 206,000 cases at its peak in 1921. In the middle of the decade, however, the US government licensed the newly available vaccine and the number of cases plummeted.

Diphtheria is now rare in industrialised countries, where infants are routinely given the diphtheria/tetanus/pertussis vaccine. However, epidemics have broken out in post-Soviet countries in the 1990s,

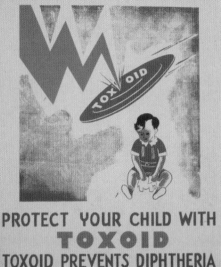

Above: Chicago Department of Health poster from the late 1930s, advertising a diphtheria vaccine for children.

and today diphtheria is still found worldwide. In 2017 a panel of WHO experts described diphtheria as a 'forgotten disease' in large parts of the world and said it needed global attention. Their research showed that progress in reducing its incidence had stalled over the previous five years, at around five thousand cases a year.

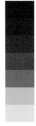

Global incidence rate of
diphtheria in 2016

3,000–3,500
2,500–2,999
1,000–2,499
500–999
100–499
10–99
1–9

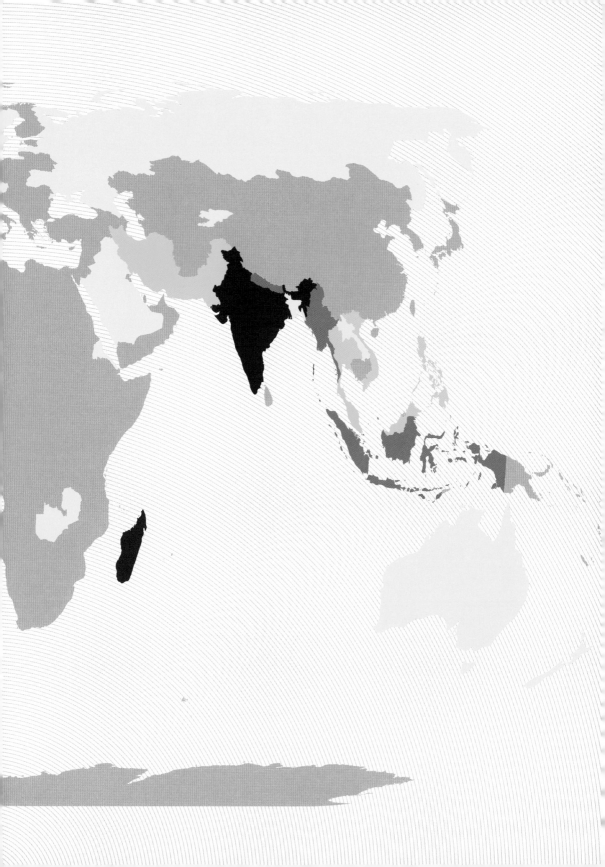

Influenza

ıιιιιιιιιιιιιιιιιιιι

Causal agent	Several strains of virus, with new strains emerging
Transmission	Mainly respiratory but also through contact with objects or surfaces
Symptoms	Fever, cough, sore throat, runny nose, muscle aches, headaches, fatigue
Incidence and deaths	Up to 650,000 deaths a year worldwide from respiratory diseases linked to seasonal flu
Prevalence	Worldwide, with the constant risk of a new pandemic
Prevention	Vaccination, but not always effective and protection is short lived. Infected cases isolated if detected early on. Advice for general population on avoiding infection during an outbreak.
Treatment	Antiviral drugs
Global strategy	Multi-factored, including surveillance to detect first signs of an epidemic and rapid response to contain it

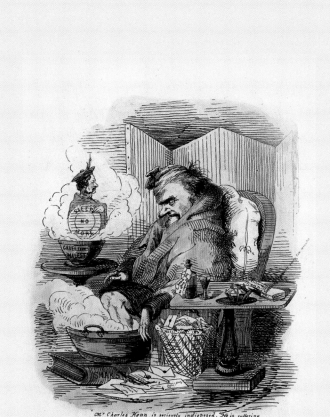

"Mr Charles Kean is seriously indisposed. He is suffering
from the effects of overwork and consequent nervous exhaustion
complicated by an attack of influenza."
Vide public Press.

Nineteenth-century caricature of the
British actor Charles Kean suffering from
the effects of influenza.

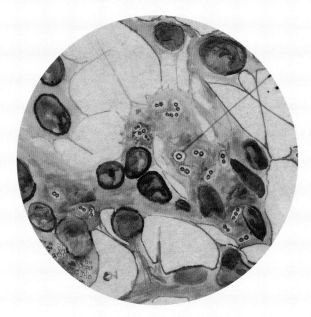

Above: Depiction of a lymph sinus,
during the 1918 influenza pandemic.

The influenza pandemic that swept the world in the autumn of 1918 killed more people than the First World War. Estimates put the death toll at around fifty million.

The event was even more extraordinary in that it came from such an unexpected source. Until then, flu had been seen as something unpleasant rather than frightening. People rarely died from it, and those who had were largely the very young, the old and those with weakened immune systems. But in 1918 that suddenly changed. For the first time, fit young adults died in droves.

Who was patient zero?

Some historians have blamed one unfortunate individual for the whole massive global tragedy. Private Albert Gitchell, a mess cook at a US army base in Kansas, stands accused of being 'patient zero' – in other words, the first person to fall sick in an epidemic. How Gitchell himself caught the infection, no one has ventured to explain.

On 11 March 1918, the soldier complained of a sore throat, headache and fever. Within hours, the infirmary was full of soldiers with the same symptoms and a month later, the medical officer had to requisition an aircraft hangar to accommodate all of his patients. Meanwhile, those men who seemed to be healthy were sent over to Europe to fight, some presumably harbouring the infection.

The Private Gitchell theory makes for a good story but not all experts are convinced. An alternative hypothesis is that the pandemic began in 1917 at the main transit camp for the British

Expeditionary force in Étaples in northern France. The camp has been described as the ideal cauldron for producing a new influenza virus, because large numbers of people, pigs and fowl were living in close proximity.

Although human beings are the main reservoir for the virus, other mammals such as pigs (swine flu) and birds such as chickens (avian flu) are also a source for some human types. The infection spreads mainly through the air when people are crowded together in enclosed spaces, and because the virus can survive for some days outside a host, it can also be spread by contact with infected surfaces such as door handles. This explains why people who nowadays work in offices or use public transport frequently, for example, are more likely to get flu.

Regardless of how the 1918 flu started, soon the pandemic was killing millions on every continent, its virulence and speed of attack causing terror worldwide. The Russian dancer Léonide Massine, giving a performance at the Coliseum in London, described how he was terrified that he would catch flu because he had to lie down on the stage wearing nothing but a loincloth 'while the cold penetrated to my bones'. He survived the ordeal and awoke the next morning in good health, only to arrive at the theatre and discover that the policeman who usually stood at the entrance, 'a hulk of a man', had died in the night.

Influenza has been described as a 'sly, nimble, deceptive sort of disease'. Sly because it infects so many people that, although only a small percentage die, these deaths add up to large numbers, and also because, unlike many other infectious diseases, it gives its victims only short-term immunity. At the height of the pandemic, there have been points at which most of the world's population was infected, although in some people the disease was subclinical – in other words, they had no symptoms.

Earlier outbreaks of flu

Influenza was probably well-established in the human population by around 5000 BC when people in some parts of the world, such as China and the Middle East, began living together and herding animals.

The Greek physician Hippocrates is thought to have described influenza in the fifth century BC, but after that there are no clear records until the fifteenth and sixteenth centuries when reports began coming out of Europe. In the summer of 1510 a disease broke out in Modena in Italy. A chronicler wrote:

> there appeared an illness that lasts three days with a great fever, and headache and then they [the victims] rise … but there remains a terrible cough that lasts maybe eight days, and then little by little they recover and do not perish.

Not long afterwards large-scale epidemics appeared to hit the continent, with an outbreak in 1580 identified as the first definite pandemic, spreading to Africa, Asia, Europe and North America. There were at least three more pandemics in eighteenth-century Europe and several epidemics, two of them extensive. An outbreak in 1781–2 is thought to have hit two-thirds of the population of central Italy and three-quarters of that in Britain. And disease also spread widely in North America, Latin America and the Caribbean.

The pattern continued into the nineteenth century. In 1889 influenza

Spread of the 1918 Spanish flu epidemic
- Focal points of the first wave
- Focal points of the second wave

Spread of the first wave

Spread of the second wave

	March 1918		September
	April		October
	May		November
	June		December
	July		January 1919
	August		Date unknown

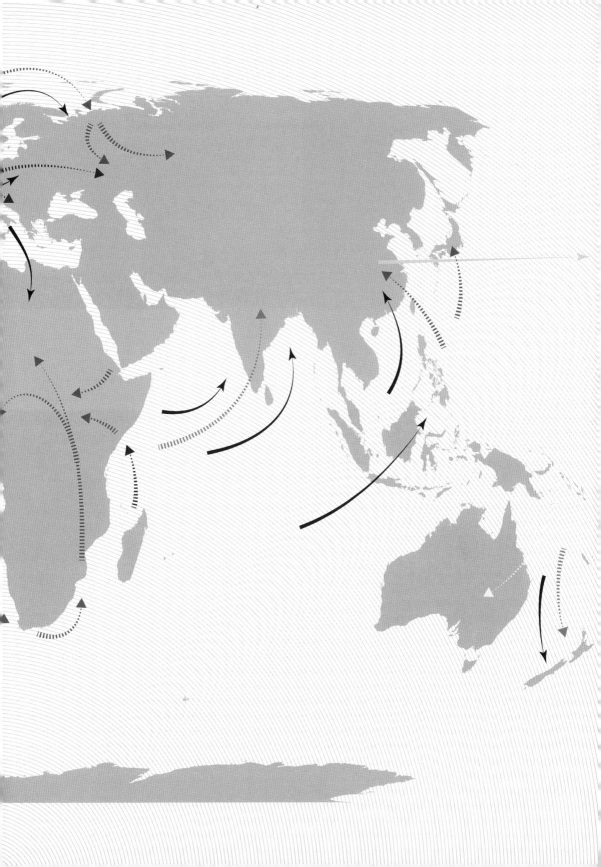

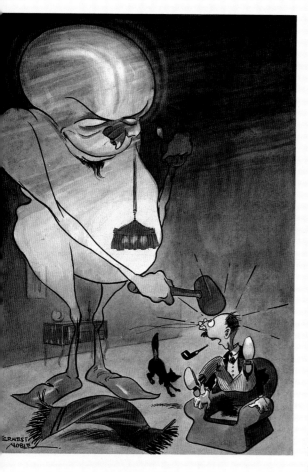

Above: Drawing of a monster representing an influenza virus, hitting a man over the head as he sits in his armchair, c. 1918.

man's disease'. Mortality rates – the number of deaths during a particular incidence or period – were quite low, as in previous outbreaks, but because of the large numbers of cases, the total number of deaths was high: at least 250,000 people in Europe and twice as many across the world.

Spanish flu

The 1918 episode was known as the Spanish flu, not because it was thought to have originated in Spain or because its ravages were any worse there, but because of the timing. The First World War dominated the agenda for the combatants, while at the same time censorship restricted reporting of any news that might damage morale or make a country appear vulnerable. In Spain, however, which had stayed neutral, there were no such constraints.

At first the flu seemed to be following its usual pattern, with high morbidity rates – the number of infections during a particular incidence or period – but fairly low mortality. In the autumn, however, that changed. A second wave of disease hit hundreds of millions of people and killed millions. It subsided towards the end of the year but then returned yet again the following winter and spring. By now about half of the deaths were of people between twenty and forty years old.

In the southern hemisphere, the timing was slightly different, as were the casualty rates. As a continent, Australia enjoyed a natural form of quarantine and the government also introduced strict screening. The impact of these factors is hard to assess, but calculations in 2002 put South Africa's death rate at fifteen times higher and the United States' at two-and-a-half times higher than Australia's.

attacked Europe from the east, earning it the name Russian flu. From here, ships carried it across the Atlantic to the United States. Two months later, it was in Canada, Brazil, Argentina and Uruguay before moving on to Singapore, Australia and New Zealand. Soon it was widespread across Asia and Africa. In parts of Africa, the infection became known as a 'white

In 1920, the disease broke out again across the world. The mortality rate was again high but not as bad as in 1918–19.

Under the microscope

Little progress was made in understanding the infection in the 1920s because microscopes were too basic and influenza was thought to be solely a disease of human beings, so no work with laboratory animals was done. By the 1930s, however, it was known that animals such as pigs and ferrets could get flu, opening up new paths for research, while the new electron microscope allowed scientists to see the flu viruses. They found that the outside surface of the virus changes radically several times in a century, so few human beings have any protection against this new subtype of virus and a pandemic explodes.

In the 1930s, three viruses responsible for influenza were identified, with the 'A' virus being responsible for the major pandemics. Although these pandemics are caused by changes in the virus, what triggers those changes is still a mystery. Like many viral infections that affect the respiratory system, influenza occurs mainly in winter. It also tends to break out in epidemics every year and in pandemics around every ten to forty years.

On into the twenty-first century and scientists continue to debate why the 1918–19 pandemic proved such a killer. One theory is that in this outbreak, the virus was often combined with a bacterial infection, which produced a deadly form of pneumonia. Another hypothesis is that this particular virus caused a massive overreaction by the body, resulting in inflammation and swelling that caused the victims to choke.

More recent outbreaks

In 1957, a new strain of virus appeared in China, causing the pandemic known as Asian flu. The infection spread rapidly across the world, westwards via the Trans-Siberian Railway into European Russia, and by sea from Hong Kong to Singapore and Japan. It reached the Indian subcontinent in May, Western Europe and both US seaboards in June, Australia and Africa in July and the UK in September. England and Wales saw around six million cases in the first twelve weeks. The infection was first concentrated in northern England but then the focus shifted south, and within two weeks, influenza was widespread throughout southern England and Wales.

In Bradford, a small outbreak within a Pakistani community was reported ahead of the main wave, probably due to an infected visitor from Pakistan. Local GPs attributed the fast spread of the disease to the Pakistani custom of visiting the sick in large numbers. 'Double peaks' like this, with a small outbreak within a defined community preceding the main outbreak were also reported among steel workers in Sheffield and coal miners in Barnsley.

Today, morbidity and mortality rates have reverted to their pre-1918 levels, with young fit adults once again at far lower risk. Influenza is still a global disease, however, and the A virus retains its potential to cause an epidemic similar to the 1918–19 outbreak. No one knows where or when the next dangerous strain will emerge and prediction is made particularly hard because human beings exchange flu viruses with both wild and domesticated mammals and birds. In China, where people and pigs live side by side in countless villages across the country, new strains are thought to be spawning all the time.

Spread of the 1957
Asian flu epidemic

First Wave, 1957
■ Probable origin
● February–May
● June–September
○ October–December

Second Wave, 1957–58
■ Probable origin
● October–January

Probable direction of migration

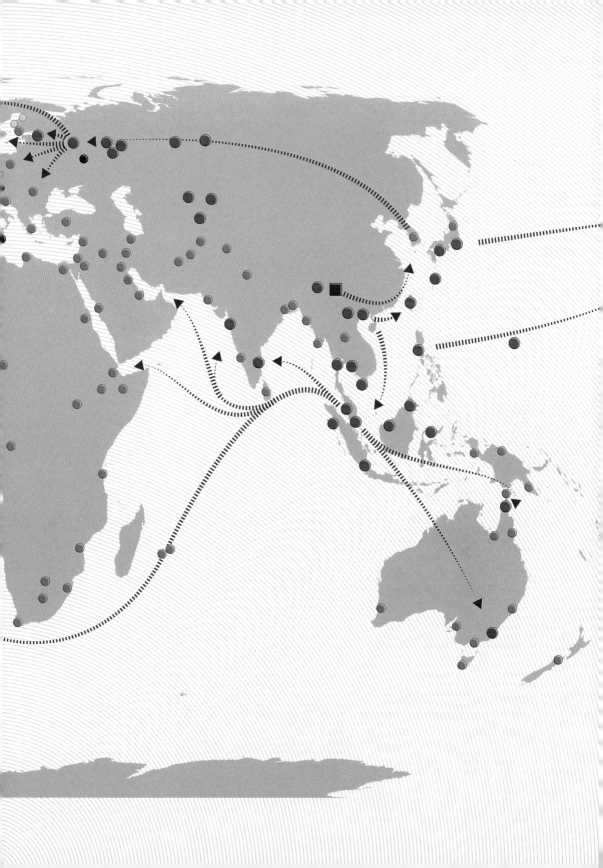

Leprosy

ıııııııııııııı

Causal agent	Bacterium *Mycobacterium leprae*
Transmission	Long thought to be through direct contact with a patient but respiratory route now believed more likely
Symptoms	Skin nodules, ulcers, thick, dry or stiff skin, loss of eyebrows and eyelashes, numbness, muscle weakness and eye problems
Incidence	Around 250,000 people diagnosed in 2017
Prevalence	Endemic in some parts of the world, mostly Africa and Asia
Prevention	No vaccine but the infection is hard to catch
Treatment	Combination of antibiotic drugs
Global strategy	The World Health Organization (WHO) goal is to eradicate the disease, with a target of zero new infections in children by 2020. Key interventions include early detection of cases and better quality of, and access to, healthcare for marginalised populations.

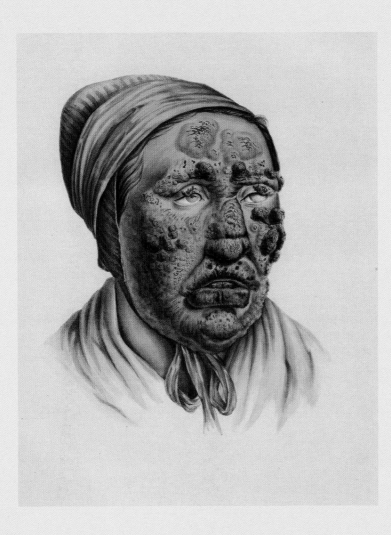

*Nineteenth-century illustration of
a woman with leprosy from a
Norwegian book on the disease.*

The term 'leper' conjures up a horrible image. A pitiful, disfigured creature wanders the streets shaking a bell and crying 'unclean'. People cross the road to avoid him. Not surprisingly, 'leper' has become a term widely used to describe any kind of outcast.

Cursed by disease

Epidemic diseases have long been seen as divine retribution – HIV and the resulting AIDS is a modern-day example – but leprosy, or Hansen's disease as it is now known, holds a special place on the punishment list. The Hebrew Bible has several references to God punishing an

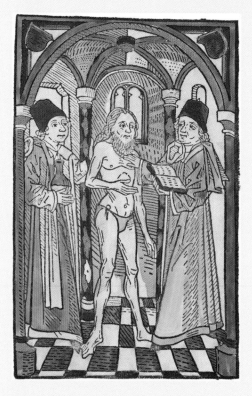

Above: *'The Leprosy Man', a woodcut from* Das Buch der Natur *(The Book of Nature), 1482.*

individual with a dose of what is assumed to be leprosy, on one occasion even telling an offender that the disease 'shall cleave unto thee and unto thy seed for ever'.

Leprosy, however, is not hereditary: it is a slow, progressive disease, caused by the bacterium *Mycobacterium leprae* or *M. lepromatosis*, found mostly in tropical countries. The pathogen can grow in the body without causing any symptoms for up to twenty years, which makes it hard to discover how an individual became infected.

Because for centuries the disease was seen as a curse rather than a medical condition, the victim was left to the priest rather than the doctor. The Bible's Book of Leviticus sets out in some detail how a leper was to be dealt with, which informed attitudes for centuries:

> his clothes shall be rent and his head bare and he shall put a covering upon his upper lip and shall cry 'Unclean, unclean'. And all the days wherein the plague shall be in him he shall be defiled; he is unclean; he shall dwell alone; without the camp shall his habitation be.

There is little room then for equivocation.

Medieval England, however, had none of the laws against lepers that prevailed in many countries, where victims were deprived of their rights in matters such as marriage and inheritance. The only such piece of legislation in England was a decree in 1346 banning lepers from London. The reasons behind it are not clear but the measure might have been in response to a specific incident or situation. The decree accuses lepers of being, at best, indifferent to the risks they pose to their fellow citizens and, at worst, of deliberately spreading the disease 'some of them endeavouring to contaminate others with that abominable blemish that, so to their own wretched solace, they may have the more fellows in suffering . . .'

They were doing this, the statute says:

> by way of mutual communications, and by the contagion of their polluted breath, as by carnal intercourse with women in stews [brothels] and other secret places, detestably frequenting the same, do so taint persons who are sound, ... to the great injury of the people dwelling in the city.

But victims were not always treated cruelly. Some people saw the suffering of lepers as similar to that of Christ, which meant that they were closer to God. In twelfth-century England, for example, lepers were often well cared for, usually by religious orders or in hospitals known as lazar houses. At the time of the London ban in the fourteenth century, attitudes changed, partly because of the horrors of plague and the Black Death, but by then the disease was on the wane in Europe, perhaps because the population had acquired some immunity.

Going back through time

Tracking diseases back through history has always been a tricky business. With only partial records and vague accounts of symptoms to go on, it can be hard to know which condition is being described. And particular confusion surrounds leprosy because many of its symptoms mimic those of other skin conditions, including fungal infections, such as the disfiguring disease favus.

The nineteenth-century dermatologist George Thin wrote of leprosy:

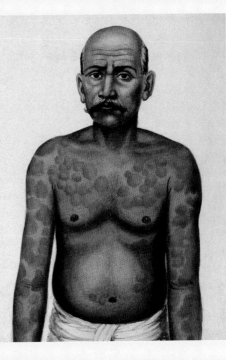

Above: *Painting of a man suffering from the early stages of skin leprosy, during the reacting phase.*

> That a distinct malady ... is recognised at all by the Jewish writers and by the Egyptians shows that there existed then, as now, one particular disease which stood out from all the other ailments ... by the severity of its symptoms, its incurability and by its grossly disfiguring and mutilating character.

Thin, however, was making a dubious claim when he referred to 'a distinct malady' in the Jewish and Egyptian records. There is nothing distinctive about leprosy in the early writings.

Some historians claim that the Greek physician Hippocrates described leprosy in the fifth century BC, and the disease may also be mentioned in ancient records

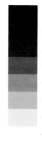

Approximate dates of
leprosy epidemics
throughout history

2,000–62 BC
1st–3rd C
4th–6th C
7th–9th C
10th–12th C
13th–15th C
16th–18th C
19th–20th C

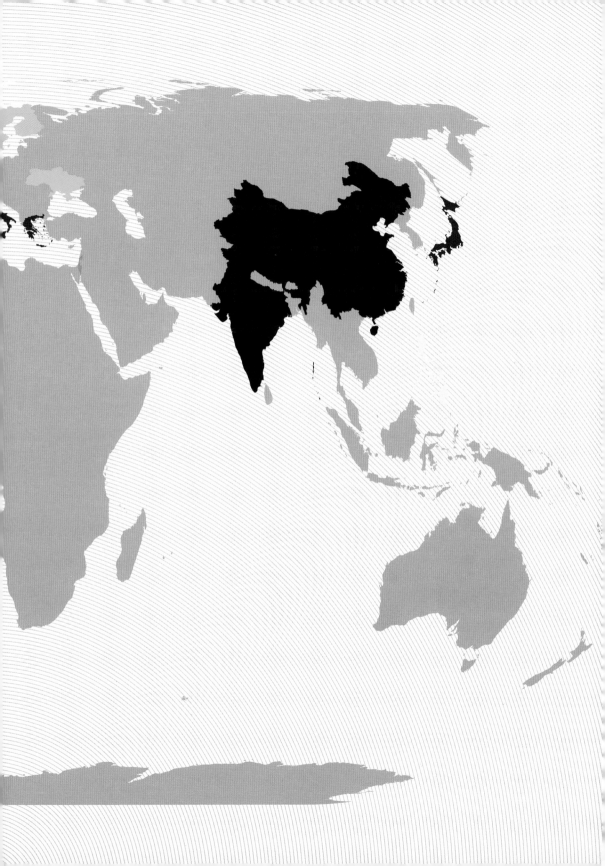

from the Middle East, India, China and Rome. A description in the third-century BC Chinese text, the 'Feng Zhen Shi', is a strong contender. The document lists leprosy under skin disorders and includes among its symptoms damage to the nasal septum (the wall between the nostrils), which is sometimes a feature.

There is some agreement that the tenth-century AD Persian physician Avicenna gave an account of the disease, but many of the references to what is called leprosy in the Bible, including the instructions for dealing with sufferers in the Book of Leviticus, are thought to refer to other skin complaints.

In 2005, researchers retraced the journey of the leprosy bacterium and concluded that the disease originated in either East Africa or the Near East, from where colonists, explorers and traders introduced it into West Africa and the Americas. From West Africa, the eighteenth-century slave trade took the disease to the Caribbean, Brazil and probably other parts of South America, the researchers report. They pointed to the many cases of leprosy in the American Midwest in the eighteenth and nineteenth centuries, which coincided with the arrival of Scandinavian settlers at a time when a major epidemic was under way in Norway.

Wild armadillos in the US state of Louisiana are naturally infected with the leprosy bacterium, but the researchers found that they also harbour the European/North African strain of the pathogen, indicating that they had been contaminated by human sources. Armadillos might, in turn, be able to spread the disease to humans but the risk is said to be very low. In this same 2005 study, the researchers refused to rule out an ancient animal origin for *M. leprae* in human beings but suggested that insect bites might have been involved.

In 2009, more evidence emerged. The remains of a man buried near the Old City of Jerusalem were dated to AD 1–50, and tests showed that he suffered from leprosy. That same year, another team reported finding the disease in the bones of a middle-aged man in India that dated as far back as 2000 BC. They said if the leprosy bacterium evolved in Africa, the disease possibly migrated to India in the third millennium BC when there was substantial contact between the Indus Valley Civilization (between north east Afghanistan, Pakistan and north west India), Mesopotamia (part of West Asia around the Tigris–Euphrates river system) and Egypt.

Strategies to eliminate leprosy

In the nineteenth century, a leper colony was set up on one of the smallest, most sparsely populated of the Hawaiian Islands. The records are hazy but suggest that at least eight thousand people were forcibly removed and quarantined there from the 1860s to around 1960s. Almost all were native Hawaiians.

In 2015, sixteen of those patients, aged from seventy-three to ninety-two, were still alive and six were still living on the island. The quarantine had been lifted in 1969, more than twenty years after an effective treatment became available, but some residents could not face leaving the isolated world that had been their home for so long.

Leprosy used to be thought of as highly contagious but, in fact, it is hard to catch and requires prolonged close contact with someone with untreated leprosy for many months. It is still not known how the disease spreads. The original theory that it spreads by direct contact with an infected person is now being replaced by the idea that it is transmitted through the respiratory route, when the sick person coughs or sneezes and the healthy person breathes in the infected droplets.

In 2000, the WHO removed leprosy's status as a global public health threat. Overall, the risk of getting Hansen's disease is very low for any adult because more than 95 per cent of the world's population is now naturally immune. There is no vaccine against Hansen's disease but today it is easily curable. Early treatment prevents sufferers from developing disabilities and so screening in high-risk areas is important.

However, the disease remains endemic in parts of the world: in 2017 about 250,000 people across the world were diagnosed with leprosy and 2 million were permanently disabled by it. Between 2011 and 2015, the vast majority of cases (94 per cent) occurred in just fourteen countries: seven in Asia, including India and Bangladesh; six in Africa, including Democratic Republic of Congo, Ethiopia and Madagascar; and in Brazil in South America. Each country reported more than one thousand new cases a year. The United States, by comparison, saw around 150 to 250 new cases a year. The WHO has set up a strategy for a leprosy-free world that includes a target of zero new infections in children by 2020. Of a total of 216,108 newly diagnosed cases in 2016, 18,472 (almost 9 per cent) were children, some of whom were already showing signs of disability.

As well as working to eliminate the disease, the WHO is also trying to remove the stigma which, the organisation says, means that adults still face terrible social

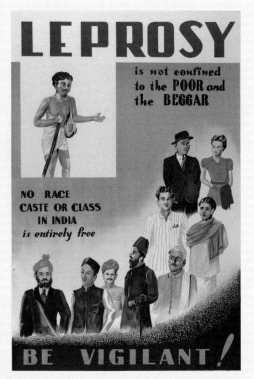

Above: *Indian poster about leprosy, highlighting the non-discriminatory nature of the disease – part of an awareness-raising initiative from the 1950s.*

barriers and children are bullied and denied education. India, for example, has sixteen laws discriminating against people with leprosy, including the disease being grounds for divorce. Patients in many parts of the developed world were encouraged or forced to live apart until well into the twentieth century. This stigma is preventing people from coming forward for diagnosis and treatment and so hampering efforts to eliminate the disease, particularly among vulnerable groups, such as migrants, displaced people and those who are ultra-poor and hard-to-reach by health services.

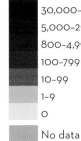

New cases of leprosy
reported during 2016

30,000–135,485
5,000–29,999
800–4,999
100–799
10–99
1–9
0
No data

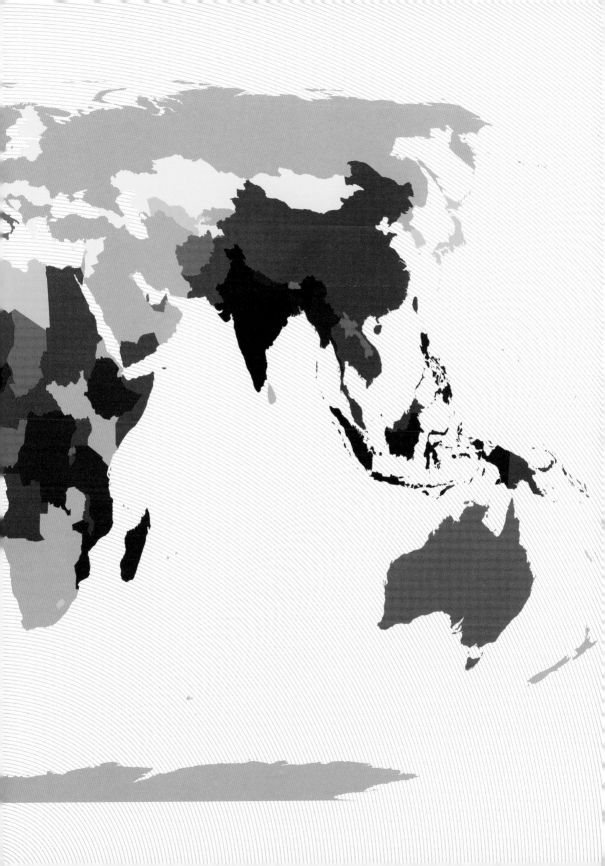

Measles

||||||||||||||||

Causal agent	Virus of the type paramyxovirus
Transmission	Respirary, highly contagious
Symptoms	Fever, runny nose, cough, red eyes and sore throat, followed by a rash over whole body
Incidence and deaths	Estimated 90,000 deaths in 2016
Prevalence	Worldwide
Prevention	Vaccination with the combined measles, mumps and rubella (MMR) vaccine
Treatment	No specific treatment for the virus but drugs for symptoms such as fever and muscle pain
Global strategy	World Health Organization Global Vaccine Action Plan (GVAP) has a goal of eliminating measles by or before 2020

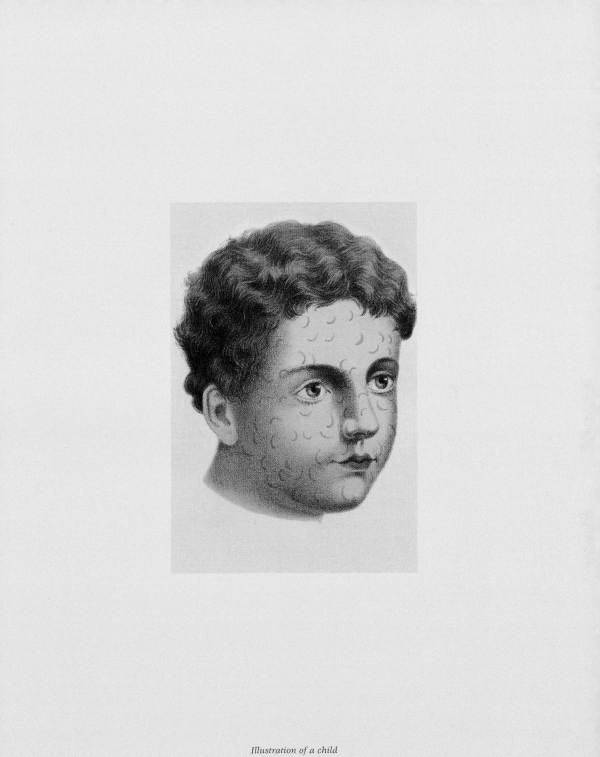

Illustration of a child
suffering from measles, c. 1912.

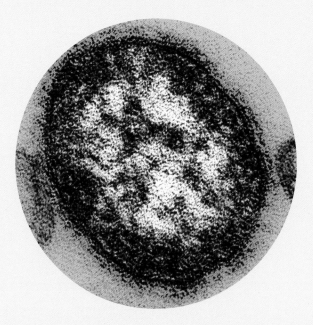

Above: *Microscopic image of a measles virus particle.*

In 1492, when Christopher Columbus set foot in the New World, the explorer is thought to have brought with him a batch of deadly diseases, of which measles proved to be one of the most fatal. A theory for its ferocity is that the new pathogen devastated the native populations because they had no previous exposure to it and therefore no immunity, but some historians disagree.

Introducing disease to the vulnerable

The event was a dramatic, though not unique, example of how adventurers, colonists and traders were carrying infections around the world to regions where they had previously been unknown. And this was not a one-way street: when the carriers returned to their own countries, they brought new pathogens with them.

In the sixteenth century, the Spanish introduced measles, along with smallpox, to the Caribbean, Mexico and Central America. Together, the two infections hit Central America and Peru so hard that some historians suggest this was why fairly small numbers of conquistadores were able to subjugate the entire Aztec and Inca peoples.

Measles, which affects only humans and monkeys, is normally passed through direct contact and through the air. The measles virus, MeV, infects the respiratory tract, then spreads throughout the body. It is highly contagious, has caused millions of deaths over thousands of years and is particularly virulent when introduced into a new population, as the New World experience showed.

Where the population does have some immunity, mortality rates are quite low, around one in five thousand cases – however, babies under one year, malnourished children and those with weak immune systems are at much higher risk. Twentieth-century research in West Africa suggests that overcrowding also exacerbates the disease, which might account for its high mortality rate among destitute children. Those living in crowded conditions might suffer badly simply because they have a heavier exposure to the virus, or viral load. And they are also likely to be exposed to some chronic infections such as tuberculosis (TB) at the same time that damages their ability to fight acute diseases like measles.

A virus with a long history

MeV is thought to have gained a foothold among humans in the Middle East somewhere between 3000 and 8000 BC, when people first began living together in large populations and herding animals. The virus is related to those that cause canine distemper and bovine rinderpest (the latter once killed entire herds of cattle but was eradicated in 2011), so it probably jumped species from animals to human beings at some point.

Below: Boys suffering from measles (left); scarlet fever (middle); smallpox (right), c. 1880.

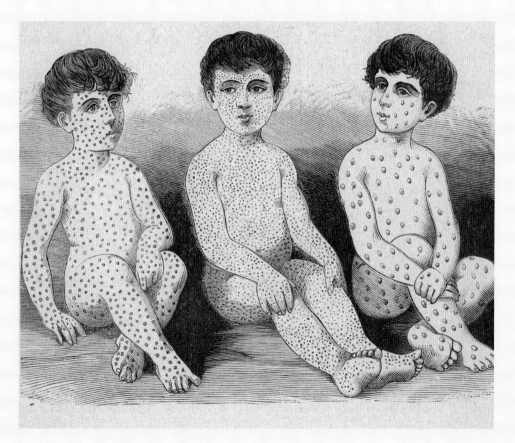

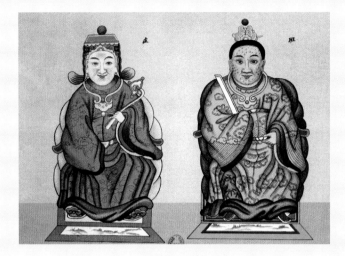

Left: *Chinese gods of disease: Tcheng Chen, the Chinese god of measles (left); Pan Chen, the god of smallpox (right), taken from* Recherche sur les Superstitions en Chine *(Research on Chinese Superstitions) by Henri Dore, Shanghai, 1911–20.*

As measles and smallpox both spread fast and produce rashes and sores, the two were confused for hundreds of years. The fourth-century Chinese alchemist Go Hung made what is said to be the first known attempt to distinguish between them, followed three hundred years later by Aaron, a Christian priest in Egypt. However, credit for the first detailed work on their identification is usually given to the tenth-century Persian physician Muhammad ibn Zakariya al-Razi, or Rhazes.

Despite the infection's long history, the first records of what are more clearly identified as measles epidemics emerged only in the eleventh and twelfth centuries. The name comes from a Middle English word for 'blemish' or 'pustule' but its earlier name, 'morbilli', is from the Italian for 'little disease', to distinguish it from 'morbus', or 'plague'.

Island populations

The poignant story of a young king and queen of Hawaii shows the power of the infection in people with no previous exposure. The couple came to London in 1824 seeking an audience with King George IV. Within weeks, virtually the entire royal party went down with measles. About seven to ten days earlier – the typical incubation period for the disease – the group had visited the Royal Military Asylum, home to hundreds of soldiers' children. Within the month the king and queen were dead.

At that time measles was unknown in Hawaii, but this changed dramatically in 1848 when the country was struck by a series of epidemics of different diseases, starting with measles and whooping cough. Measles, thought to have arrived either from Mexico or California, swept through the islands, killing between 10 per cent and 33 per cent of the population. There then followed a wave of outbreaks through the nineteenth century, followed by an epidemic in 1936–7 that caused 205 deaths.

Two years before measles hit Hawaii, it struck another island group. More than 75 per cent of the 7,782 residents of the Faroes, between Iceland and Norway in the North Atlantic, became sick, and more than one hundred people died. The Danish physician Peter Ludwig Panum studied how the epidemic behaved, tracking its spread from village to village. In a classic piece of 'on the ground' epidemiology, he discovered that none of the older people who had measles during an outbreak back in 1781 had been attacked this time. His discovery would later become key to developing a vaccine.

In 1875, another royal family on a Pacific Island group was affected by measles. The Royal Navy ship HMS *Dido* arrived in Fiji, bringing King Cakobau and his two sons back from a state visit to New South Wales. The monarch was recovering from measles which he had caught in Sydney and then passed on to his sons. Over the next ten days the royal family entertained sixty-nine chieftains and their entourages, around five hundred people in all. At the same time, passengers with active measles also arrived on two more ships and were allowed to land. The resulting epidemic killed forty thousand people, according to the colonial governor, up to one-third of the population. The

shocked islanders believed that the disaster was due either to poison or bewitchment.

However, the London Epidemiological Society published a witness account that suggested the high death toll was not directly due to the disease alone:

> The attacks are so sudden and complete that every soul in a village will be down at once and no one will be able to procure food or, if obtainable, to cook it for themselves or others. The people have died from exhaustion and starvation in the midst of plenty.

Protection against infection

After the First World War, measles deaths dropped significantly in the UK. Medical historians have speculated about the reasons but one theory points to some wartime welfare reforms and perhaps also to women becoming the main wage earners in working families, increasing their children's share of the family food supply.

In 1954, Thomas C. Peebles, a Second World War bomber pilot-turned-doctor, isolated the measles virus, and in 1963 a safe, effective vaccine became available. During 2016, about 85 per cent of the world's children received one dose of measles vaccine in their first year, up from 72 per cent in 2000. From 2000 to 2016, vaccination prevented an estimated 20.4 million deaths worldwide, making the vaccine 'one of the best buys in public health', according to the World Health Organization (WHO).

Even so, the disease still presents a major risk. In 2016 it killed 89,780 people, and in 2017, and again in 2018, the WHO warned that measles was once again spreading across Europe in those countries where vaccination rates had dropped. At

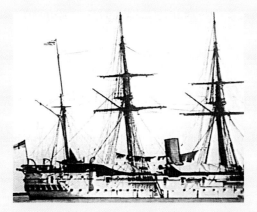

Above: *Starboard side view of the HMS* Dido, *c. 1871. The ship is painted white for tropical service.*

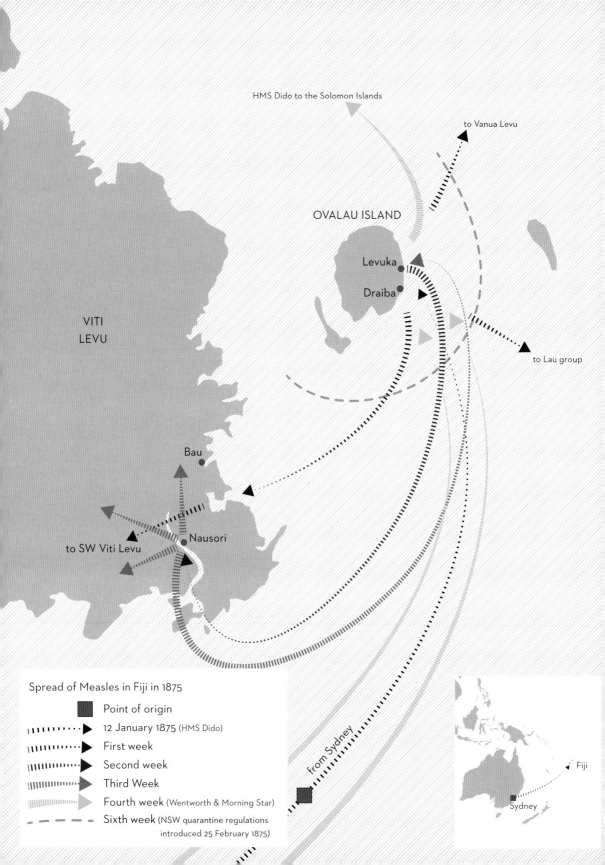

HMS Dido to the Solomon Islands

to Vanua Levu

OVALAU ISLAND

Levuka

Draiba

to Lau group

VITI
LEVU

Bau

to SW Viti Levu

Nausori

Spread of Measles in Fiji in 1875

■ Point of origin

▶ 12 January 1875 (HMS Dido)

▶ First week

▶ Second week

▶ Third Week

▶ Fourth week (Wentworth & Morning Star)

– – – Sixth week (NSW quarantine regulations
introduced 25 February 1875)

from Sydney

Fiji

Sydney

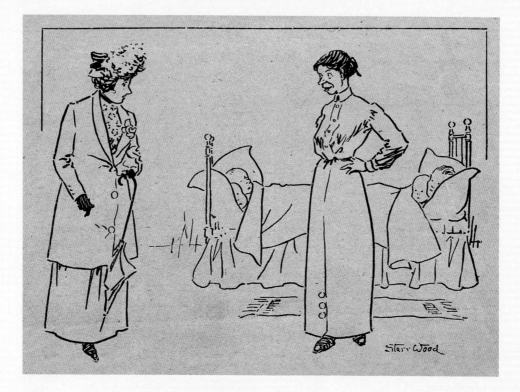

least 95 per cent of a population needs to be vaccinated to achieve 'herd immunity' to measles. Herd immunity is where there is a large enough pool of protected people to prevent the disease from spreading.

In 2017, cases quadrupled from those in 2016 to more than 21,000 across Europe. Thirty-five people died. Fifteen European countries were hit, particularly Romania with 5,562 infections, followed by Italy with 5,006 and Ukraine with 4,767. The WHO's regional director for Europe described the situation as 'a tragedy we simply cannot accept'. The high incidence in Romania was blamed on a combination of a shortage of vaccine, an anti-vaccine movement and difficulties in reaching marginalised groups of people, but the resurgence of measles in the rest of Europe

Above: Sketch in which a mother tells a nurse there's no risk of infection because her children with measles are at the opposite end of the bed to her healthy ones, 1915.

was blamed on the growing strength of anti-vaccine movements.

Behind the anti-vaccine movement

A big setback for immunisation in Europe and the United States came in 1998 when the respected British medical journal *The Lancet* published a paper by Andrew Wakefield, a gastroenterologist. He claimed he found a link between the combined measles, mumps and rubella (MMR) vaccine and autism and bowel disease in children. His claim was false and Wakefield was later struck off the UK Medical Register;

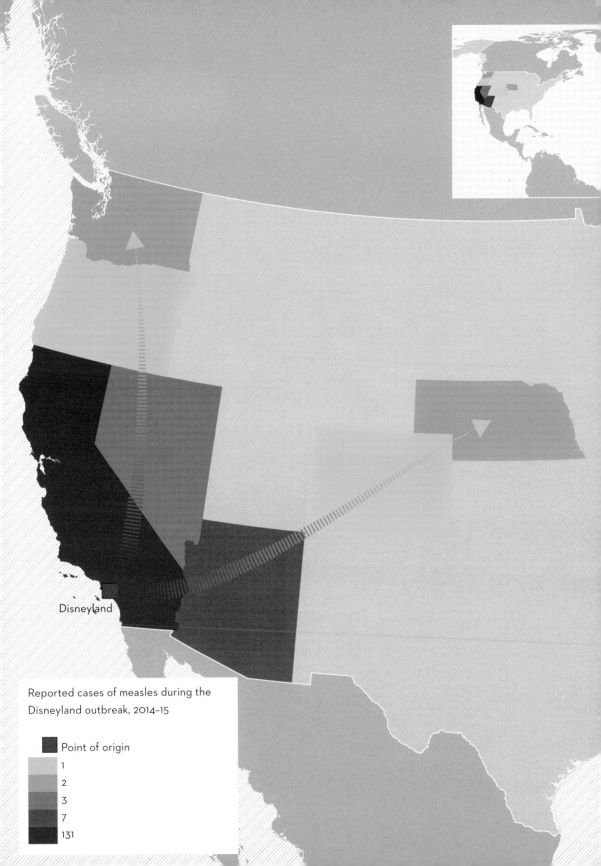

Disneyland

Reported cases of measles during the
Disneyland outbreak, 2014–15

Point of origin
1
2
3
7
131

however, the repercussions of his actions are still being felt.

In 1997, the year before Wakefield's paper was published, measles vaccination rates in the UK stood at more than 91 per cent. They started to fall in 1998 and in 2003–4 were down to just 80 per cent nationally, with rates even lower in some areas. The dramatic drop in vaccination rates between 1998 and 2004 resulted in a rise in measles cases. In Swansea, between November 2012 and July 2013, for example, there were more than 1,200 cases, the largest number in Wales since the triple vaccine was introduced.

As a result, some countries such as France and Italy made some vaccines mandatory. In the United States, where measles also made a come back, the state of California was no longer recognising parents' personal beliefs as a valid reason for not vaccinating their children. The WHO announced plans for a public awareness campaign and for improving vaccine supplies, stating: 'This short-term setback cannot deter us from our commitment to be the generation that frees our children from these diseases once and for all.' Since 2004 the take-up began climbing again, reaching about 90 per cent in 2013.

Recent outbreaks

In 2000, the US government announced that it had eradicated epidemic measles but, of course, this did not prevent imported cases. In 2015, the country saw two outbreaks with more than six hundred cases. One hit the unvaccinated Amish community in Ohio after a missionary returned from the Philippines where an epidemic was raging. The other was a multi-state outbreak linked to the Disneyland amusement park in California. The experts failed to identify the source but suspected the infection was brought in by an overseas visitor. They did discover that the virus type was identical to that which caused the the Philippines epidemic.

In Vietnam, in the spring of 2014, an estimated 21,639 suspected measles cases were reported, with 142 measles-related deaths. In a remote part of northern Myanmar, at least forty children died in an outbreak in August 2016 that was probably caused by lack of vaccination in an area where the health infrastructure is poor. Under the WHO GVAP, the organisation's six regions each have set goals to eliminate measles by or before 2020.

Scarlet fever

IIIIIIIIIIIIIIIII

Causal agent	Bacterium from the streptococcus group, usually *streptococcus A*
Transmission	Respiratory and through contact with infected items such as towels and bed linen
Symptoms	Sore throat, fever and distinctive red skin rash
Incidence and deaths	No global figures but largely eliminated as a major killer
Prevalence	Recent upsurges in cases in some countries including England
Prevention	Precautions when in contact with an infected person
Treatment	Antibiotics as well as drugs to reduce the fever

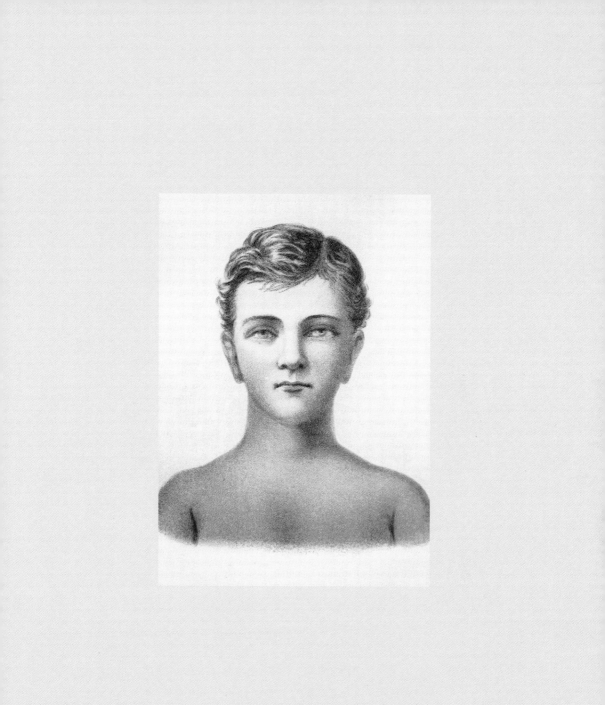

Illustration of a child
with scarlet fever, c. 1912.

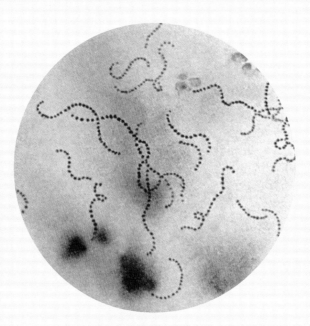

Above: *Illustration of the* Streptococcus pyogenes *bacteria, which causes scarlet fever.*

The plague has been banished. It is unlikely that cholera will in this country ever attain the severity it has had in the past. The outbreaks of smallpox are now limited. We have banished typhus from our jails. A like success cannot, however, be claimed for scarlet fever.

So, in 1879, wrote William Stephenson, professor of midwifery and of diseases of women and children at the University of Aberdeen.

In fact, by then death rates for scarlet fever, or scarlatina, were on their way down in Britain and Western Europe, albeit from a considerable peak. The number of deaths from scarlet fever, mostly in children, nearly doubled in Britain from 1836 to 1840, and the toll continued to rise in a series of epidemics over the next three decades. By the 1870s, the disease had become the most deadly of all infectious diseases among children.

A double threat to impoverished children

In 1870, scarlet fever killed 32,543 children in England and Wales. Although the large numbers of deaths were partly because the disease was more widespread, it had also become more dangerous. And the outbreak of 1858–9 also coincided with the return of diphtheria, another throat condition that is particularly deadly to children.

In the 1880s, the disease remained fairly common, but the mortality rate began to edge back down as the infection became milder. The risk though was still very real. In 1910, Ramsay MacDonald, the MP who was to become the Labour Party's first prime minister, lost his young son, David. The boy was recovering from scarlet fever when he contracted diphtheria, and the double assault proved too much for his system. Six months later, Ada Salter, a friend of David's mother, Margaret, lost her eight-year-old daughter, Joyce to scarlet fever. The Salters were socialists who had chosen to live and work in Bermondsey, a deprived part of London. Joyce had already survived two bouts of the infection but the third overwhelmed her.

It had been well-established that the risks of infection from many diseases were far higher for children living in slums. In the previous year, 1909, Bermondsey had 411 cases of scarlet fever and eight deaths, compared with Hampstead's 101 cases and no deaths. But no one was exempt: the MacDonalds lived in a wealthy Bloomsbury square.

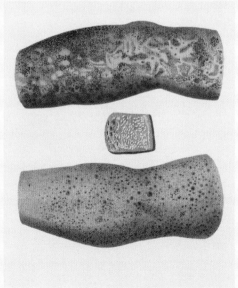

Above: *Handcoloured copperplate stipple engraving showing the effects of scarlet fever by John Pass from John Wilkes'* Encyclopedia Londinensis, *1822.*

Similar symptoms, different diseases

Scarlet fever is caused by *Streptococcus pyogenes*, one of a group of bacteria responsible for many different diseases in human beings, ranging from mild to life-threatening infections. Different strains of *S. pyogenes* also vary greatly in the severity of the disease they cause. Russia and Eastern Europe continued to suffer from a particularly toxic form of scarlet fever well into the twentieth century.

When, where or how scarlet fever first emerged to infect human beings and the route it took across the world remain a mystery. It is largely a disease of temperate climates where it occurs mainly in winter. Descriptions of a similar-sounding illness date back almost 2,500 years to the ancient Greeks. It is thought to have been around at low levels in Britain for centuries but because, like diphtheria, it causes a sore throat, swollen tongue and raging fever and mostly attacks children, the early history of the two diseases is muddled.

Both are highly contagious and spread mainly through droplets in the air; in the early twentieth century, they carried a similar mortality rate of around 15 to 20 per cent. As late as the 1840s, many doctors still thought that scarlet fever and diphtheria were different forms of the same illness, but the pathogens responsible are quite different, as are some of the symptoms. The rough, scarlet-red rash that resembles sandpaper is particular to scarlet fever and there is no suffocating membrane as in diphtheria (see page 15).

To add to the confusion, scarlet fever's red rash has also led to difficulty in distinguishing it from measles. The seventeenth-century English physician Thomas Sydenham tried to throw some light on the problem: 'The whole skin is

Cases of scarlet fever recorded in
Europe in WW2

1939
1944 (reduction in cases)
1944 (increase in cases)

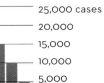

25,000 cases
20,000
15,000
10,000
5,000

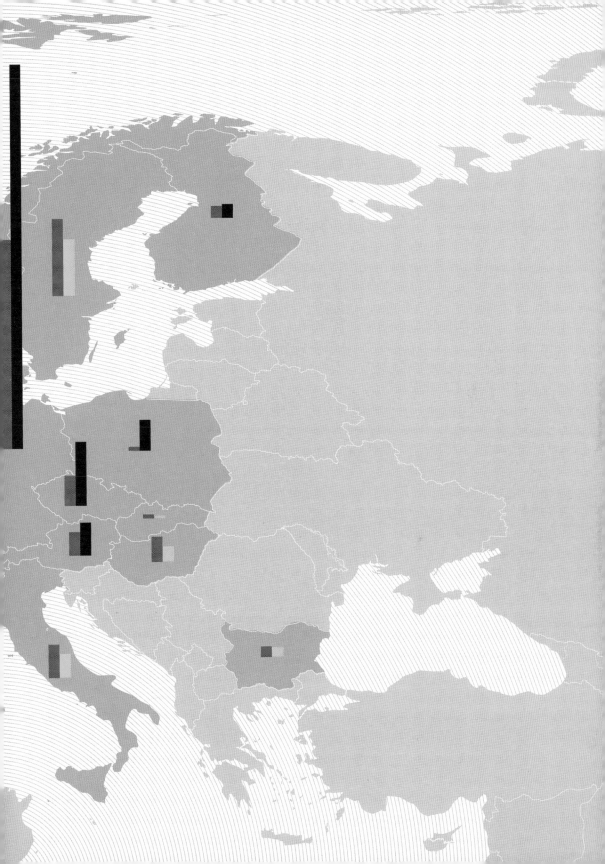

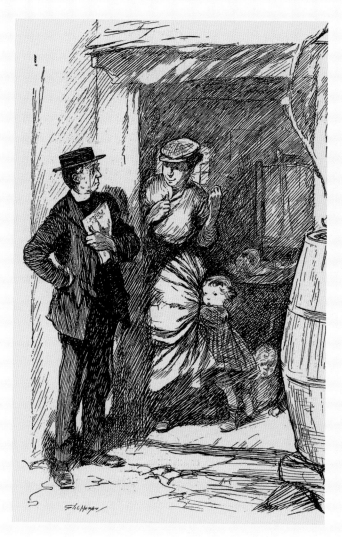

covered with small red spots, which are more numerous, larger and redder but not so uniform as those which constitute the measles.'

Credit for the first clear description of the symptoms is usually given to the tenth-century Persian physician Muhammad ibn Zakariya al-Razi, or Rhazes, followed in the sixteenth century by the Italian doctor Giovanni Ingrassia, who defined it as a specific disease during an epidemic in Palermo in 1553 and described its fiery rash. Ingrassia called it rossalia, but in 1676 Sydenham gave it the Latin name *febris scarlatina*, or 'scarlet fever', a reference to the colour of the rash.

Suddenly a major killer

Initially, in the seventeenth century, scarlet fever appears to have been fairly rare and mild, usually seen in small local outbreaks, perhaps affecting just a few families. Sydenham certainly didn't seem to regard it with any great concern, describing it as 'nothing more than a moderate effervescence of the blood, occasioned by the heat of the preceding summer'. He advised doctors not to over treat it with blood-letting or enemas but rather to tell the patient to refrain from eating meat or drinking 'all kinds of spirituous liquors' and recommended they stay in their room but not necessarily in bed.

But at the same time that Sydenham published his work, scarlet fever had started to manifest itself in larger outbreaks in towns and cities across Europe, reaching Denmark in 1677 and Scotland in 1684, as well as in the United States in 1735. These outbreaks became steadily more regular and more deadly possibly due to a change in the bacteria. In Britain, the death rate rose from 2 per cent of cases in the late eighteenth century to 15 per cent in 1834. In some cities, mortality even reached more than 30 per cent, making it one of the deadliest diseases of the time. In 1901, it killed the grandson of the American philanthropist John D. Rockefeller, which gave a new impetus to the millionaire's existing plans to open a research centre for infectious diseases.

In the early twentieth century, a milder strain appeared once again and by the mid-1920s scarlet fever deaths in England and Wales had fallen to around nine hundred a year. The picture was the same in Australia. The first cases there were recorded in Tasmania in 1833, followed by Victoria and New South Wales in 1841, and from then on until about 1910 the disease was a major cause of death, but then the death toll began to fall.

In England, during the Second World War, thousands of London schoolchildren were evacuated to the countryside to escape the Blitz. Public health experts warned that the large-scale dispersal of children from a city with a history of epidemic diseases such as scarlet fever might spread these infections among the country children, who had little previous exposure. And indeed, the incidence of scarlet fever and diphtheria rose heavily during the two main phases of evacuation, 1939–40 and 1944–5, in the fourteen counties that received the London children.

No longer a threat?

While there is still no vaccine for scarlet fever, penicillin in the 1940s, followed by other antibiotics more recently, have largely eliminated it as a major killer across the world. Even so, the disease in its milder form still breaks out from time to time. In China, cases rose from 15,234 in 2002 to 62,830 in 2015, and an epidemic in 2011 affected 67,358 children in China, Hong Kong, Macao, Taiwan and South Korea. In Hong Kong, nearly two thousand cases were reported in the first eleven months of 2017, up nearly 60 per cent when compared to the same period in 2016.

England has seen steep increases since 2014, and in 2016 the government agency Public Health England reported a slight increase in severe infections, announcing that the situation was being monitored closely. In February 2018, doctors in England were once more alerted to an 'exceptional increase' in scarlet fever. The reasons for these upsurges are not understood, although a decrease in immunity in the general population, a stronger strain of bacteria and a combination of both have been suggested as possible causes.

SARS

IIIIIIIIIIIIIIIIIII

Causal agent	Severe acute respiratory syndrome coronavirus or SARS-CoV
Transmission	Not completely understood but thought to be through close contact with an infected person, mainly through the respiratory route, and also through contact with infected surfaces
Symptoms	Influenza-like, including fever, malaise, myalgia, headache, diarrhoea and shivering
Incidence	No reports of SARS since 2004, as of mid-2018
Prevalence	Currently no cases reported but potential to break out and spread worldwide
Prevention	Fast reporting of new outbreaks, isolation of infected individuals and contacts
Treatment	No specific treatment but general antiviral drugs and treatment to support breathing, prevent or treat pneumonia and reduce swelling in the lungs
Global strategy	Worldwide surveillance to detect new outbreaks, fast reporting of cases and containment

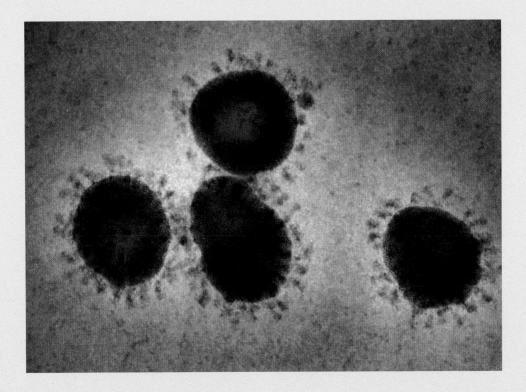

Microscopic image of the
coronavirus that causes SARS.

On 16 November 2002, a young man from a farm in the Guangdong province of South China was admitted to Foshan No. 1 People's Hospital, suffering from what seemed to be an unusual form of pneumonia. He recovered, although how and why he contracted the illness is still a mystery. Over the following weeks, more people were diagnosed with what appeared to be the same condition, but not all of them were as lucky as the farmer and several people died.

Rapid spread from the Orient

Three months later, a medical specialist who had recently treated some of the Guangdong patients went to Hong Kong to attend a wedding. As he checked into the Metropole Hotel, however, he began to feel ill. He died a few days later. In less than 24 hours, the sickness had spread to several of his fellow guests, among them a 78-year-old Canadian woman. Two days later, she flew home to Toronto, where she too developed pneumonia-like symptoms and on 5 March she died. Over the coming weeks, as a media circus descended on the city, around four hundred people in Canada experienced similar symptoms, twenty-five thousand Toronto residents were put into quarantine and forty-four people died.

Among the guests at the Metropole was Johnny Chen, a Chinese–American businessman. He was taken sick on a flight to Vietnam and was admitted to a hospital in Hanoi, where he died, but not before the illness had spread to medical staff and other patients. At the time, the Italian doctor Carlo Urbani, a World Health Organization (WHO) expert on communicable diseases, was based in Hanoi. He received an urgent call from the hospital and went to investigate the outbreak. Urbani concluded that they were dealing with an entirely new infection and

Below: Chest x-ray of a person affected by SARS.

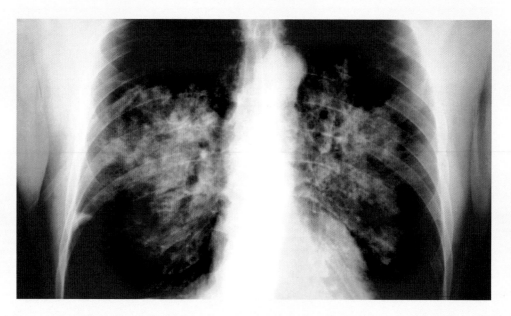

he alerted the WHO accordingly. He, too, then fell ill and died.

In mid-March 2003, under the headline 'Killer bug reaches Europe', *The Sunday Times*, a London-based newspaper, reported that more than 150 passengers flying from New York to Singapore had been quarantined in Frankfurt over fears they might have been exposed to 'a new form of pneumonia that doesn't respond to conventional treatment'. Quarantining in a time of epidemic disease is one of the oldest and most controversial of public health measures, but in the twenty-first century, faced with uncertainty and no vaccine, the authorities still resort to the practice.

By the third week of March, 350 suspected cases, 10 of them fatal, had surfaced in 13 countries, including Italy, Ireland, the United States, and Singapore. Two weeks later, the tally had risen to 18 countries, with more than 2,400 cases and 89 deaths. The WHO sent a multinational team of experts to China to investigate, while the United States added SARS to the list of diseases for which an individual could be quarantined.

International response

The WHO later said Urbani's actions allowed many new cases to be identified at an early stage and the patients to be isolated before they could infect large numbers of people. The organisation issued an alert for doctors worldwide to be on the lookout for SARS. The International Health Regulations played an important part here. First introduced in 1969 to help monitor and control cholera, plague, yellow fever and smallpox, they were revised by the WHO in 2005, following the SARS epidemic to cover new and re-emerging diseases.

Two weeks before Urbani fell ill, the Chinese Ministry of Health had reported 305 cases of what it described as 'an acute respiratory syndrome of unknown cause' in Guangdong. Five people had died. Three days later China told the WHO that the first cases had, in fact, come to light four months earlier. At the end of February, the WHO officially recognised the condition that became known as severe acute respiratory syndrome, or SARS.

The Chinese government apologised for the delay in reporting the outbreak and announced 'the immediate establishment of a national medical emergency mechanism, with emphasis placed on a public health information and an early warning reporting mechanism'. In the meantime, meat markets in southern China and Hong Kong were banned over fears that SARS could be caught by eating infected animals.

On April 22, although the number of cases started to level off, the US Centers for Disease Control and Prevention cautioned: 'We have no capacity to predict where it's going or how large it's ultimately going to be'.

As well as the risks to health, the epidemic was also having an economic impact. By the end of April tourism in Thailand was down by 70 per cent and Singapore by 60 per cent. The British Foreign Office meanwhile was advising against travel to Hong Kong, parts of China and Toronto.

A new — and fatal — coronavirus

In April 2003, researchers in Hong Kong published a paper identifying a new type of what is known as a coronavirus as a likely cause of SARS. The term 'coronavirus' comes from the Latin for 'crown' or 'halo' and refers to the crown-like spikes on the

Spread of SARS from China between
January and April 2003

January
February
March
April

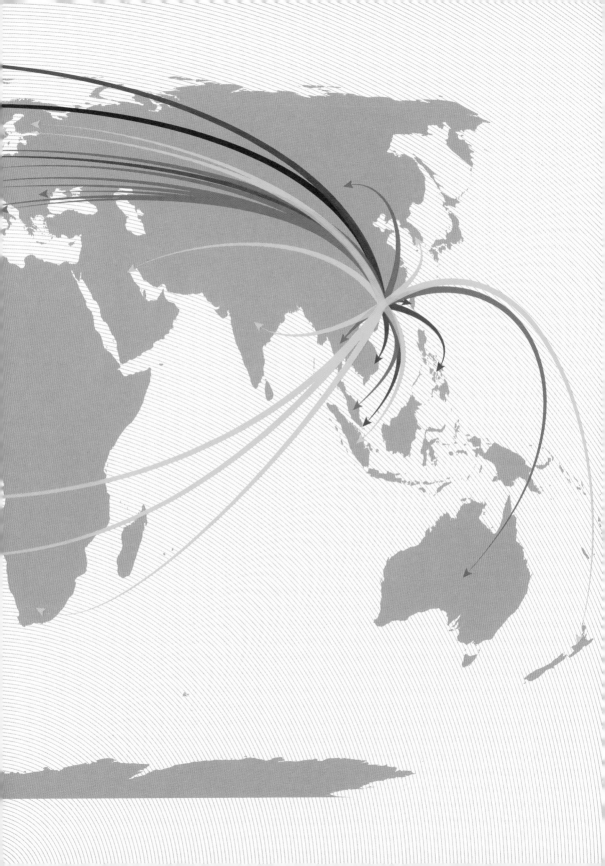

Recorded cases of SARS during
2002–3 outbreak

5,001–5,500

1,001–5,000

501–1,000

101–500

21–100

2–20

1

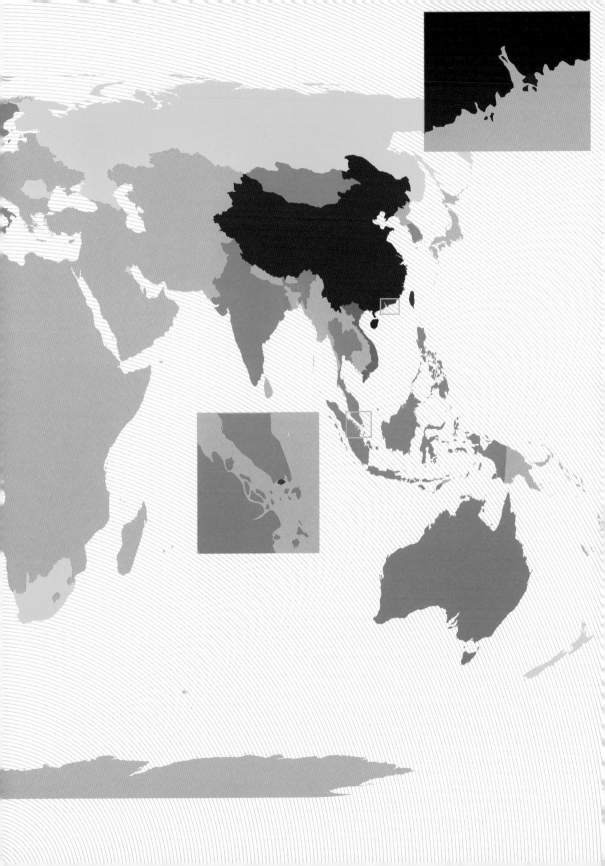

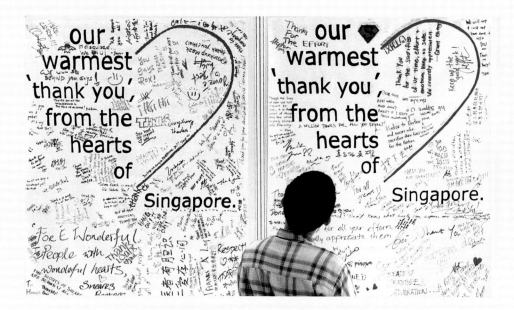

pathogen's surface. This particular coronavirus, SARS-CoV, does not appear to have been seen before in humans or in animals.

Coronaviruses are common and most, like the common cold, are not dangerous. Others, like SARS, however, can be fatal. SARS is believed to be be passed on mainly through close contact with someone who is infected, including kissing, hugging, touching, sharing eating or drinking utensils with, or being within a metre (three feet) of them. It spreads mainly through droplets in the air when the infected person coughs or sneezes. The virus can also spread when someone touches a surface or object contaminated with infectious droplets and then touches their mouth, nose or eye. It might also spread more broadly through the air or in other ways that are not yet understood.

On 23 April 2003, work started on a new 1,000-bed hospital for SARS patients on the outskirts of Beijing. The new Xiaotangsham Hospital went up fast but

Above: A tribute to the medical teams caring for the SARS patients in Singapore, 2003.

treated only 680 patients. By the end of June, it was no longer needed. The WHO gave China the all clear and in early July the organisation announced that all twenty-nine countries that had seen cases of SARS were free from the disease. The pandemic that had struck countries in North America, South America, Europe and Asia, infecting 8,098 people and killing 774, was over as quickly as it had begun.

Much is still unknown about SARS, including its origins. When researchers announced a SARS-like virus had been isolated from civet cats captured in the part of China where the outbreak began, the Chinese government began a cull, killing more than ten thousand civets as well as badgers and racoons. The Chinese horseshoe bat has also been suggested as a possible source.

The emergence of MERS

As of early 2018, there had been no reports of SARS since 2004. In 2012, however, the United States declared the SARS virus a 'select agent', meaning that it had the potential to pose a severe threat to public health and safety. That same year another new coronavirus emerged in Saudi Arabia.

A patient died in a hospital in Jeddah from acute pneumonia and organ failure. Doctors were unable to identify the pathogen involved and sent sputum samples to a laboratory in Holland, where the Middle East respiratory syndrome coronavirus (MERS-CoV) was identified as the cause of what is known as Middle East respiratory syndrome, or MERS. The illness is similar to SARS and carries a mortality rate of around 40 per cent.

By early 2018, twenty-seven countries had reported cases of MERS, including the United States, Iran, the Philippines and several countries in Europe such as the UK. About 80 per cent of all cases were in Saudi Arabia, however, where people are believed to be able to catch the disease from an infected dromedary camel as well as an infected human. MERS possibly originated in bats before spreading to camels. Cases outside the Middle East usually involve travellers who were infected in the region.

The WHO told all countries to be on the alert for MERS, whether or not they had had cases, especially where large numbers of people were coming in from the Middle East. They were also instructed to report both confirmed and probable cases, while at the same time outlining how they were dealing with them, in order 'to inform the most effective international preparedness and response'.

How and why one human coronavirus – the common cold – could have been around as a mild irritant for centuries and a new and deadly one suddenly emerged was 'a troubling question', one expert remarked after the SARS outbreak. Since then, that new and deadly one has been followed by a second.

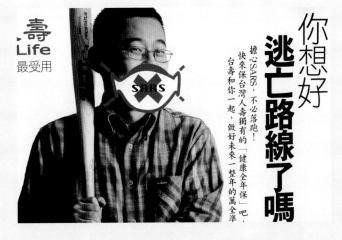

Left: *A poster warning about the SARS outbreak in Taiwan, 2003.*

Smallpox

||||||||||||||||

Causal agent	Virus of the orthopoxvirus genus
Transmission	Respiratory route and also through pus from the rash of an infected person
Symptoms	High fever and pustular rash that left permanent scars
Prevalence	Eradicated in 1979; so far the only human infectious disease to be so
Prevention	Vaccination was highly effective
Treatment	There was no proven treatment but some antiviral drugs were thought to have had some benefit

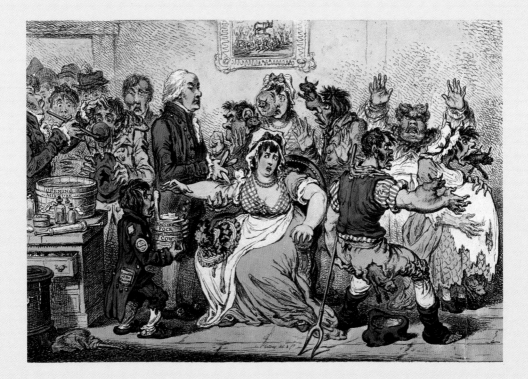

Caricature of Edward Jenner inoculating
patients, who are then shown growing cow heads
from parts of their anatomy, 1802.

An ancient illustration shows Shitala seated on a donkey, a bowl in one of her four hands. In one of many versions of the story, the Hindu goddess is told that she will always be worshipped as long as she carries lentil seeds. But as she travels with her companion, the demon of fever, the seeds somehow turn into smallpox germs, infecting everyone whom the pair encounter. Shitala, who is recognised in several Asian religions and cultures as the goddess of smallpox, is seen as both the cause and cure for the disease.

Smallpox's appearance in scripture and legend gives it a unique place among killer diseases, although others, such as plague and typhus, have proved as devastating down the centuries. But smallpox holds another, rather more inspiring, distinction: it is the first infectious human disease to be banished from the planet.

Smallpox is an acute, contagious disease caused by the variola virus. Its name comes from the Latin for 'spotted', and at the height of its virulence in the seventeenth and eighteenth centuries it was known as the speckled monster. Experts think it might have evolved from an African rodent virus around ten thousand years ago. There are two main types of variolmajor and minor. Variola major was the predominant endemic strain, and by the end of the eighteenth century it was responsible for approximately four hundred thousand deaths a year in Europe.

Civilisation: a breeding ground for disease

Humans were the virus's only natural reservoir so, without an animal carrier, the population had to reach a critical number in order for endemic smallpox to become established. When people began to living together in populations in regions such as the river valleys of Egypt, India and China they provided a breeding ground for diseases like smallpox.

The infection was airborne, spreading through face-to-face contact between an infected person and a healthy one via droplets from the nose or throat. Occasionally, however, it travelled over longer distances and was passed on through contact with objects such as a patient's bedding.

Lesions on the mummified face of King Ramses V of Egypt, who died in 1157 BC, indicate he might have been a victim of the disease and might have died from it. An early written account of a disease resembling smallpox appears in a Chinese manuscript dated 1112 BC that refers to a 'fearful plague'. However, exactly when smallpox was introduced into China is under debate and one account by the fourth-century physician Ko Hung dates it to AD 25–49.

Another possible reference comes from seventh-century India, but credit for the first clear description of smallpox is usually given to the tenth-century Persian physician Muhammad ibn Zakariya al-Razi, or Rhazes.

In the West, smallpox is under suspicion as being the epidemic that hit Athens in 430 BC, killing unknown numbers of people, and also as the so-called Antonine Plague, which felled ten thousand people in first-century Rome. This pandemic then spread across the Empire to North Africa, Western Asia and other parts of Europe, causing an estimated five million deaths.

Reports of possible outbreaks then crop up with increasing regularity in the Middle East, including in fourth-century Syria, and France and Italy may have seen an epidemic in AD 570, but the disease that hit in Japan in the eighth century has been identified with more certainty.

Increase in travel, spread of disease

Like many infectious diseases, the history of smallpox is linked to invasion, exploration, trade and the growth of civilisations over the centuries. It was introduced into Japan in the eighth century through trade with China and Korea, and Arab invaders took it to North Africa and the Iberian peninsula. Three hundred years later, it travelled with the Crusades deeper into Europe and then Portuguese colonists brought it to West Africa.

Historians have suggested that the devastation caused by smallpox and measles in the New World explain why relatively small numbers of conquistadores were able to subjugate the entire Aztec and Inca kingdoms in the early sixteenth century. In the decades after the Spaniards arrived in Peru and Mexico, smallpox deaths have been put at up to 3.5 million. In the same century the slave trade brought the disease to the Caribbean and Central and South America, while seventeenth-century Europeans brought it to North American and eighteenth-century British explorers to Australia.

In 1789, a year after the British arrived in Australia, smallpox devastated the Aboriginal population of New South Wales in just one month. By then the disease had attained an unenviable status as the most devastating of the Western world.

Unlike some other infections, smallpox was no respecter of wealth or class: victims included members of the royal families of England, France, Russia, Spain and Sweden. In 1526, Queen Elizabeth I became dangerously ill but recovered, but

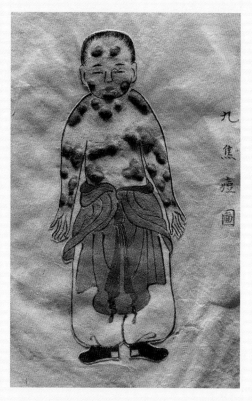

Above: *Textured watercolour illustration from a Japanese work on smallpox, c. 1720.*

in 1694 Queen Mary, wife of William III of England, died, as did Louis, the Grand Dauphin of France in 1711, along with three siblings of Francis I, the future Holy Roman Emperor, and Emperor Joseph of Austria. (Joseph reportedly promised his wife he would stop having affairs if he survived.)

In the space of one year, in 1707, smallpox wiped out around eighteen thousand of Iceland's population of fifty thousand, and later in the eighteenth century, the US city of Boston, Massachusetts was hit by eight epidemics.

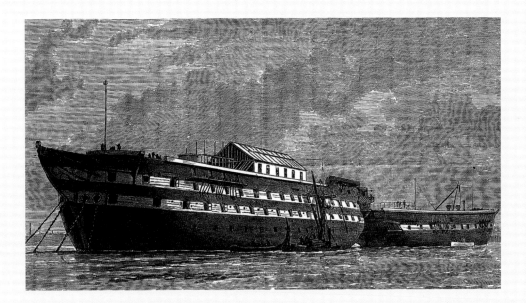

The introduction of inoculation

But as smallpox was at the peak of its powers there came a huge medical advance that would lead, not only to eventual defeat of that disease, but to the control of other deadly epidemics. Inoculation – giving a weak form of a disease to stimulate the body into producing antibodies to fight off future attacks – had been used against smallpox in Asia and Africa for centuries. It was done by taking infected matter from the pustules of a victim with a mild case of the disease and either scraping it into a cut in a healthy person's skin or letting them inhale it. The principle was sound but the early unscientific methods used could result in disaster.

In 1714, Dr Emanuel Timonius wrote to the Royal Society in London saying inoculation had been practised in what was then Constantinople (modern-day Istanbul) for forty years and was 'a happy success'. The Reverend Cotton Mather of Boston, Massachusetts then came forward with a story of his own to tell:

Above: The ships Atlas *and* Endymion *at Deptford Creek, UK, used as smallpox isolation hospitals in the 1880s.*

Enquiring of my negro man, Onesimus, who is a pretty intelligent fellow, whether he had ever had the smallpox, he ... told me that he had undergone an operation which had given him something of the smallpox and would forever preserve him from it ... he showed me in his arm the scar which it had left upon him.

Onesimus was from what is now southern Libya.

Lady Mary Wortley Montagu had an important role in making smallpox inoculation accepted in Britain. She, too, had come across the practice in Turkey. In 1721, when medical ethics left something to be desired, seven condemned prisoners in Newgate jail were offered the chance of escaping execution if they took part in an experiment. Unsurprisingly, they all agreed to be inoculated and they all survived.

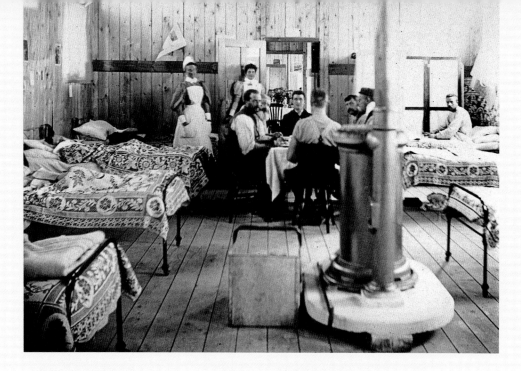

Then in 1796 the English physician Edward Jenner took the practice to a new level. Jenner grew up in rural Gloucestershire, where country people had long known that a mild disease that was common among milkmaids, known as cowpox, gave protection against smallpox. In a famous experiment, unthinkable today, Jenner inoculated his gardener's son, eight-year-old James Phipps, not with smallpox but with cowpox and then exposed him to smallpox on several occasions. Fortunately for James, Jenner was right and the boy failed to develop the disease. The practice became known as vaccination, from the Latin *vacca*, meaning 'cow'.

Despite initial scepticism, the idea took off in Britain and the knowledge spread fast. From 1804 to 1814, two million people were vaccinated in Russia.

Eradication of a disease

Steadily, country by country, region by region, smallpox was eliminated. The first country to be clear was Iceland's tiny isolated population in 1872, with the UK following in 1934 and North America in 1952. An outbreak in New York in 1947 saw the mobilisation of one of the world's largest vaccination programmes in the United States, and it is seen as a model example of public health planning and practice. When Portugal was declared free of smallpox in 1953, the continent of Europe was also free of the disease.

By the mid-twentieth century, developed countries were using vaccination and border regulations to try to stay smallpox free, but even so the disease remained a threat. In 1962, England and Wales saw two outbreaks when infected travellers arrived from Pakistan: nineteen people died in Cardiff and six in Bradford. Mass vaccination was quickly introduced.

Elsewhere, however, progress was slower. In 1960 fifty-five countries reported

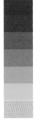

Number of cases of smallpox reported by
April during the outbreak in India in 1974

10,000–18,000
5,000–9,999
1,000–4,999
500–999
100–499
1–99
No data

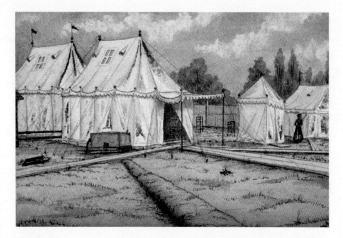

Left: *Painting of the St Pancras Smallpox Hospital, London, which was housed in a tented camp at Finchley, 1881.*

one hundred thousand cases, most of them in Africa. In 1974, fifteen thousand people died in India, but by then the disease's days were numbered. In 1959, the World Health Organization (WHO) had embarked on a global eradication campaign at the instigation of the Soviet delegate. The first efforts foundered, but an intensified programme in 1967 proved more successful and during the 1970s South America, Asia and, finally, Africa were cleared.

In 1975, a three-year-old Bangladeshi girl, Rahima Banu, became the last person in the world to have naturally acquired variola major, the most virulent of the two virus strains. She was isolated at home with a twenty-four-hour guard at the door, while health workers began going door to door, vaccinating local people, and a reward was offered to anyone reporting a smallpox case. The last case of natural variola minor was that of Ali Maow Maalin in Somalia in 1977.

Finally, in 1978, a British woman, Janet Parker, became the last person in the world to die of smallpox. A medical photographer at Birmingham University Medical School, she was working one floor above the microbiology department where researchers were working with the virus. She is thought to have become infected either via an airborne route through the building's duct system or by direct contact in the department.

In 1980, the WHO declared that smallpox had been eradicated from the entire world – the first and, as of early 2018, the only human disease to be eliminated. However, scientists wanted to keep some stocks of the virus for research. The number of holding laboratories was reduced first to four and then to two: the US Centers for Disease Control and Prevention (CDC) in Atlanta, Georgia and the State Research Centre of Virology and Biotechnology in Koltsovo, Russia.

Some argue, however, that the remaining stocks should be destroyed, saying that the scientific reasons for keeping the variola – for example, as a model for research on other viruses – are outweighed by the risks. In 2014, the CDC announced that vials containing the virus had been discovered in a cardboard box in a refrigerator at the National Institutes of Health in Bethesda, Maryland.

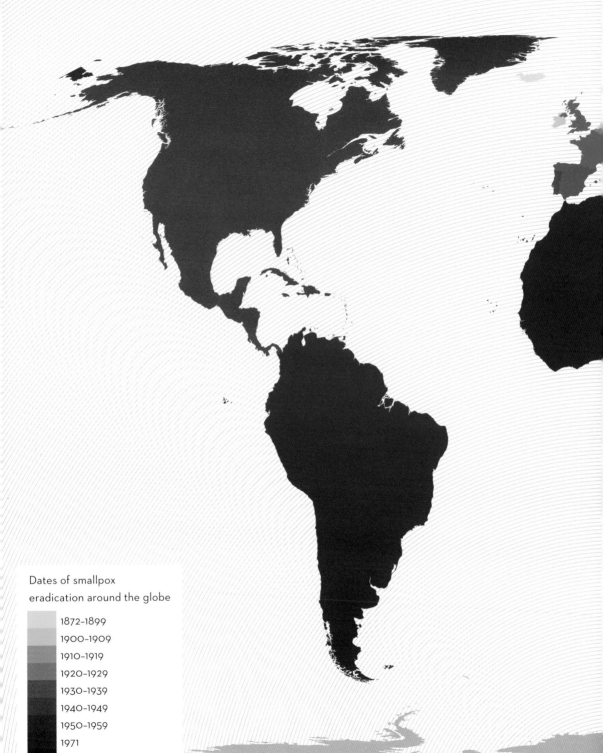

Dates of smallpox
eradication around the globe

1872–1899
1900–1909
1910–1919
1920–1929
1930–1939
1940–1949
1950–1959
1971
1975
1977
Not endemic

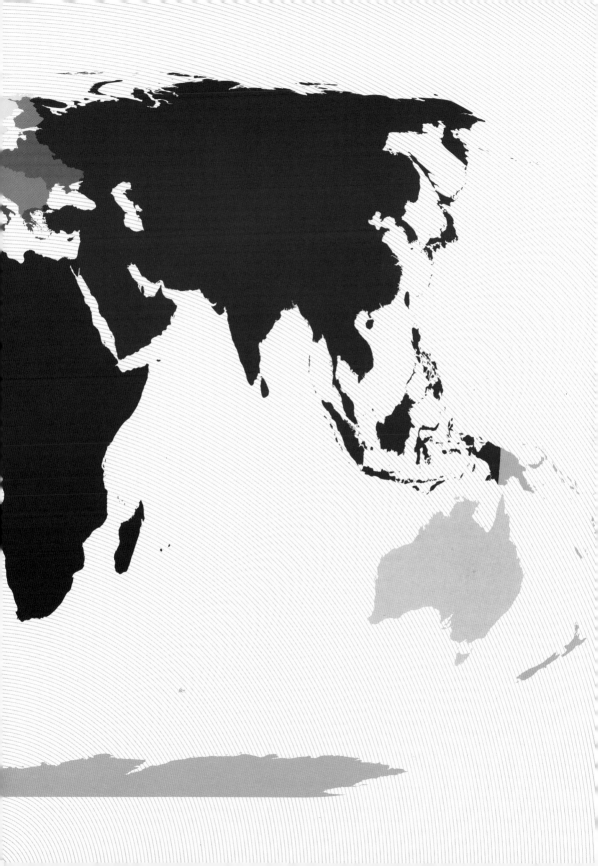

Tuberculosis (TB)

||||||||||||||||

Causal agent	Bacterium *Mycobacterium tuberculosis*
Transmission	Respiratory route
Symptoms	Active lung TB: cough with sputum and blood at times, chest pains, weakness, weight loss, fever and night sweats
Incidence and deaths	6.3 million new cases reported and 1.8 million deaths in 2016
Prevalence	Worldwide but vast majority of deaths are in developing countries, with seven including India, Pakistan and Nigeria accounting for over 60 per cent of the total
Prevention	Vaccination
Treatment	Antibiotics but drug-resistance is growing
Global strategy	The World Health Organization (WHO) aims to reduce deaths by 90 per cent and incidence by 80 per cent by 2030 which, the WHO says, requires universal health care and social protection for people in 'epidemic' countries

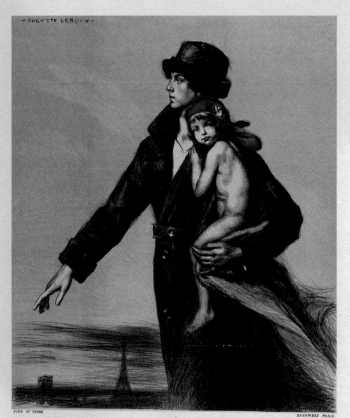

French poster promoting a campaign
against tuberculosis and infant mortality, 1918.

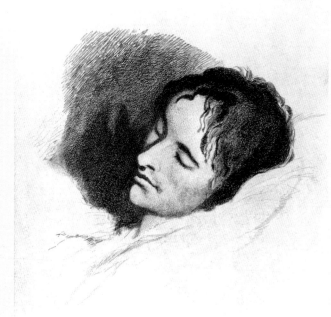

Right: Portrait of English poet John Keats on his deathbed in Rome, 1821.

The poet Lord Byron, deciding that he looked a little pale one day, is said to have announced that he would like to die from tuberculosis because women would say: 'Look at that poor Byron, how interesting he looks in dying.'

In Europe, in the first half of the nineteenth century, TB acquired a certain kudos, the terminal illness of choice for people of fashion and taste. The symptoms had much to do with it: there was none of smallpox's suppurating pustules nor cholera's loss of bowel control but a noble, tragic fading away. The scenario was an inspiration for artists and writers, notably Alexandre Dumas, the younger, in his novel *The Lady of the Camellias* and Giuseppe Verdi in his opera *La traviata*. As it happened, Byron didn't die of tuberculosis but of an unidentified fever, possibly malaria, in Greece. His fellow poet John Keats, however, did succumb at just twenty-five years old.

Gradually, a more realistic view of tuberculosis began to prevail as the disease began to spread. By the mid-1800s, it was responsible for about a quarter of all deaths in Europe. It affected all occupations and social classes but, as with most communicable diseases, it tended to go for the labourers and the washerwomen rather than the Romantic poets.

A disease of many names

Tuberculosis, or TB, is the name for a group of illnesses caused by the bacterium *Mycobacterium tuberculosis*. The disease can affect any part of the body, including the glands, kidneys, bones and nervous system, but it usually attacks the lungs – this is referred to as pulmonary TB. The illness has been known in the past by several different names, including phthisis and Pott's disease, but it was most commonly called consumption because of the way it 'consumed' its victims, wasting their bodies away.

The term 'scrofula' – mycobacterial cervical lymphadenitis – was used to describe a swelling of the lymph nodes in the neck linked to TB. For centuries people believed that scrofula could be cured by a monarch's touch, hence it also being known as the king's evil. The practice of kings and queens laying hands on patients began in England in the eleventh century under Edward the Confessor. When the German protestant George I came to the throne in 1714, however, he discontinued it, declaring it 'too Catholic'. The writer Samuel Johnson was brought to Queen Anne to be touched when he was two years old and he also had surgery on his neck, which left him badly scarred.

Humans are the main reservoir, or long-term host, of the disease, but in some parts of the world mammals such as cattle, badgers and pigs are also hosts. The organism has no natural habitat in the environment but is thought to have evolved along with its hosts over millennia. The strain *M. bovi*s mainly infects cattle, but humans can also catch what is known as bovine TB, usually through drinking infected milk.

In the nineteenth century, doctors tried inoculating people with the bovine strain to see if it would protect them against the human variety. Their thinking was based on Edward Jenner's smallpox vaccine (see page 75), which gave immunity against that disease by infecting the individual with the related, but much milder, cowpox. Unfortunately, the theory turned out to be disastrously wrong.

M. bovis wreaked just as much havoc in the human body as did *M. tuberculosis*.

History found in bones

Early evidence of the disease was found in people living in the Eastern Mediterranean around nine thousand years ago in one of the first villages to show signs of agriculture and domesticated animals. Signs have also been discovered in Stone Age skeletons and in five thousand-year-old Egyptian mummies, and the disease in its various different forms is mentioned in early Greek and Chinese texts. It is thought to have been carried to the New World by migrants from Asia, probably across the Bering Strait. Evidence, again from bones, puts the disease in North America in 800 BC and South America in AD 290.

Although *M. tuberculosis* is necessary for TB to develop, it is not the only factor involved. Age and genetics also have a part to play, as well as overcrowded living conditions, a bad working environment and poor nutrition. TB has been attacking humans for thousands of years, but it only realised its true potential as a mass killer when people began crowding together in towns and cities, breathing, coughing and spitting over each other. In the eighteenth century, large epidemics broke out around the world, hitting hardest in those countries where urbanisation and industrialisation were well underway, such as England, the United States, Italy and France.

Birth of the sanatorium

Down the ages, physicians made regular attempts to discover what caused the disease and to find a cure. The big breakthrough, however, came in 1882 when the German physician Robert Koch

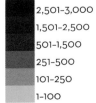

Tuberculosis incidence in high-burden
countries worldwide in 2016 (in 1,000)

- 2,501–3,000
- 1,501–2,500
- 501–1,500
- 251–500
- 101–250
- 1–100

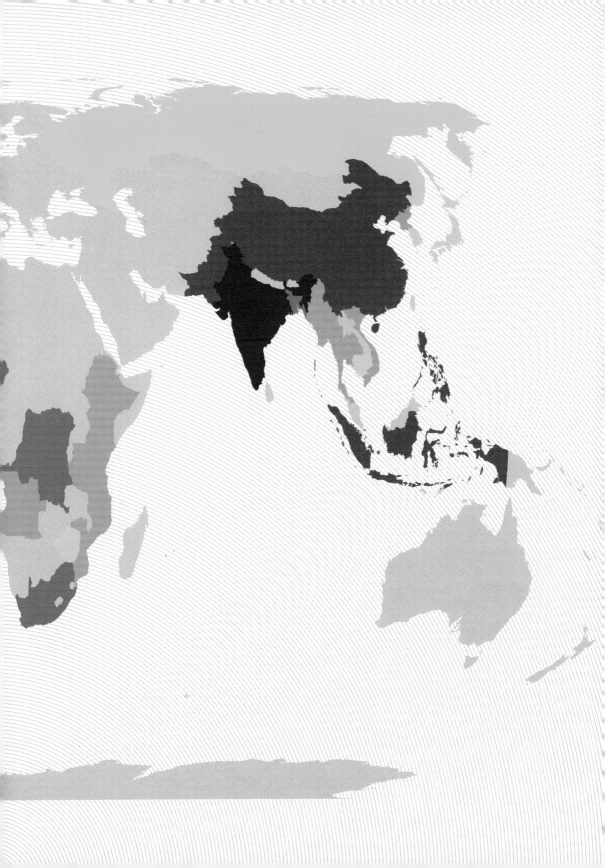

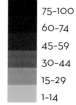

Tuberculosis death rate in 2016
(per 100,000 population)

- 75–100
- 60–74
- 45–59
- 30–44
- 15–29
- 1–14

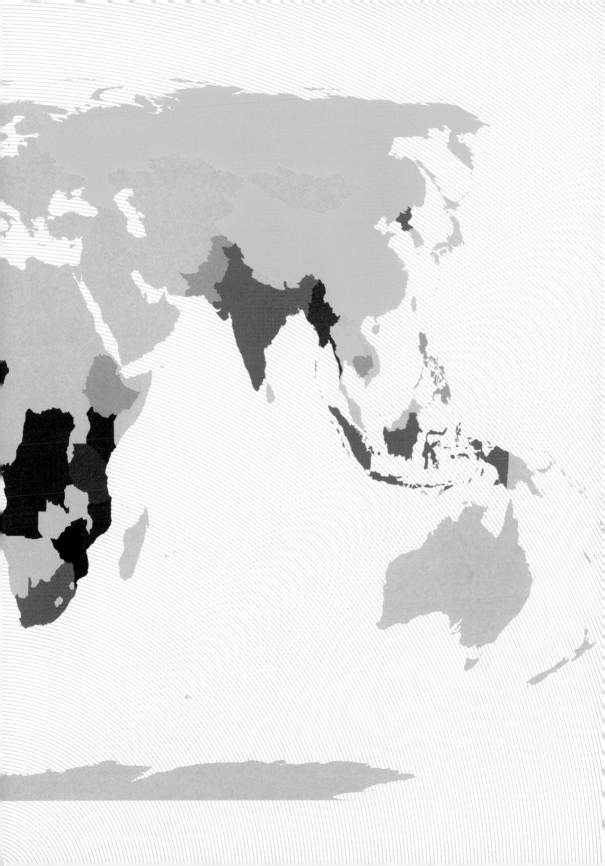

identified *M. tuberculosis*. When he announced his finding, he reminded his fellow scientists of the devastating powers of TB, stating:

> If the importance of a disease for mankind is measured by the number of fatalities it causes, then tuberculosis must be considered much more important than those most feared infectious diseases: plague, cholera and the like ... One in seven of all human beings dies from tuberculosis.

As Koch implied, by then the disease seemed to have become so familiar that it had lost the shock factor and become an accepted fact of life.

At the same time, however, a new treatment was finding favour. Doctors had noticed that some TB patients went into remission of their own accord, sometimes for the rest of their lives. No one understood why this was, but if the body had the potential to beat the disease by itself, then it made sense to strengthen it for the fight by means of a healthy lifestyle: a wholesome diet, rest, gentle exercise and, above all, fresh air. So, in the early twentieth century what was known as the sanatorium movement took off. Patients went to specialist clinics for weeks or months, living out in the open air, as pure and dry as possible, which made the Swiss Alps a favourite destination in Europe.

At first only the rich could afford it: many Swiss clinics were more like luxury spas with five-star service, gourmet cooking and entertainment. When Britain's sanatoria opened, they offered more basic care and some were aimed at working people, with charities funding treatment. Here, the emphasis was on education rather than gourmet meals. Patients would be taken for a month or so, instructed in healthy living and then sent away with a schedule of work and rest, a diet sheet and instructions on cleanliness. A certain moral undertone crept in, the implication being that working-class patients had encouraged their own ill health with their dirty, dissolute ways.

For those with a back garden, there were instructions on how to build a labourer's version of the Swiss clinic – a shelter or open shed in the garden. Even so, the vast majority of the poorest patients were still left at home or sent to the workhouse infirmary to recover or die.

The sanatorium movement was followed by the solaria treatment, again with the emphasis on a healthy outdoor lifestyle. The Swiss doctor Auguste Rollier opened a new type of Alpine clinic with south-facing balconies, sliding-glass walls and retractable roofs. Each morning, patients were wheeled out onto the balconies and gradually exposed to increasing doses of sunlight. Suntans quickly became the rage.

Preventive measures

Gradually into the twentieth century, tuberculosis began to decline in the developed world but the trend had little to do with fresh air or sunshine. First, the discovery of a diagnostic test meant victims could be identified and isolated early on, helping to stop the spread of the disease. The symptoms of active TB can be mild for months, during which time the untreated victims can infect around ten to fifteen others over the course of a year.

Slum clearance programmes in the inner cities, which reduced overcrowding, also helped cut infection rates, while

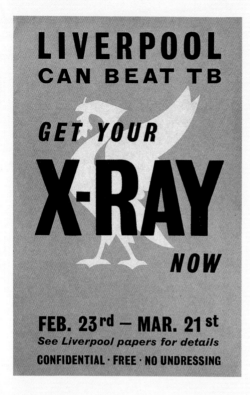

LIVERPOOL
CAN BEAT TB

GET YOUR

X-RAY

NOW

FEB. 23rd – MAR. 21st
See Liverpool papers for details
CONFIDENTIAL · FREE · NO UNDRESSING

Above: *X-ray campaign against tuberculosis in Liverpool, UK, c. 1960.*

the pasteurisation of milk and culling of infected cattle reduced the incidence of bovine TB. The greatest benefits, however, came from the development of a vaccine – although the efficacy of what is commonly known as the BCG is now debated – and effective drugs, that is, antibiotics.

In 2014, the WHO announced a strategy to reduce deaths by 95 per cent and to cut new cases by 90 per cent by 2035. TB is still to be found in every part of the world, but the incidence has fallen sharply in developed countries. Even so, it remains one of the top ten causes of death worldwide, killing 1.7 million people in 2016. More than 95 per cent of those deaths were in developing countries: seven countries, including India, Pakistan and Nigeria, account for 64 per cent of the total. TB is also a leading killer of people with HIV. Without treatment, 45 per cent of people with TB die from the disease, but for those who are HIV-positive, the rate rises to almost 100 per cent.

Not everyone infected with TB becomes sick. In 2017, about 25 per cent of the world's population had latent tuberculosis, which means they were infected but not ill and not able to transmit the disease. However, they did have a 5–15 per cent lifetime risk of developing the active disease, and certain groups, including people with HIV or suffering from malnutrition or who smoke tobacco, are at much higher risk.

The fight to keep TB under control continues even in countries where the disease is now relatively rare. In 2013, the UK government began culling badgers, which were said to play a key role in spreading bovine TB to cattle. Animal rights campaigners bitterly opposed the policy and expert opinion was firmly divided over its effectiveness. The programme continued, however, with 19,274 badgers culled in England in 2017.

After the great scientific advancements that helped to bring the devastating wave of tuberculosis under control in the twentieth century, a new threat has emerged: that of multidrug-resistant TB. In 2016, there were 600,000 new cases that were resistant to the previously most effective first-line drug, and 490,000 of those cases were also resistant to more than one drug. WHO says this is a public health crisis and a health security threat.

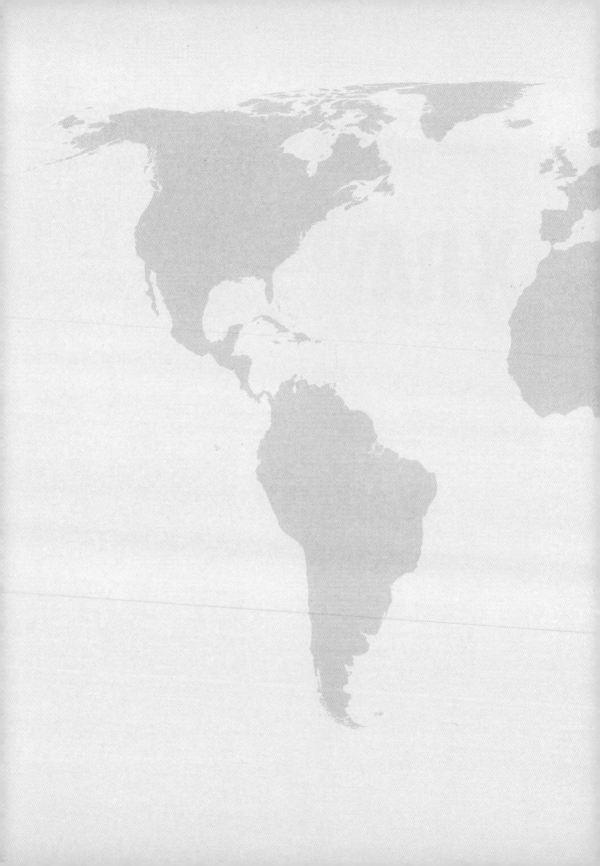

SECTION 2
WATERBORNE

Cholera

|||||||||||||||||

Causal agent	The bacterium *Vibrio cholera*
Transmission	Predominately waterborne
Symptoms	Severe diarrhoea, nausea, vomiting, stomach cramps, muscle spasms
Incidence and deaths	Estimated 1.3 million to 4.0 million cases and 21,000 to 143,000 deaths worldwide.
Prevalence	In 2016, major epidemics struck Haiti, the Democratic Republic of Congo, Somalia, the United Republic of Tanzania and Yemen. Virtually non-existent in developed countries
Prevention	Provision of clean drinking water and efficient sewers; oral vaccines in high-risk areas
Treatment	Oral rehydration in mild cases; rapid treatment with intravenous fluids and antibiotics in severe cases
Global strategy	The World Health Organization (WHO) aims to reduce cholera deaths by 90 per cent by 2030. Strategy includes: specialist treatment centres and better access to clean water, effective sanitation and waste management; good hygiene and food safety practices; and public information.

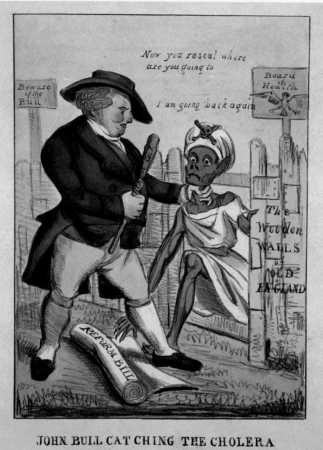

JOHN BULL CATCHING THE CHOLERA

Satirical lithograph of John Bull (the personification of Britain) defending his country against the invasion of cholera, c. 1832.

Cholera has probably been endemic to India for centuries. Ancient Indian texts describe a disease that is almost certainly cholera, and there are accounts by sixteenth-century Portuguese colonists of a mysterious sickness with similar symptoms. However, it was not until the nineteenth century that cholera was identified as a specific disease and scientists began to understand how it was spreading. By that time cholera had ravaged most of the globe, killing millions.

Spreading from the subcontinent

The disease first emerged from the Sundarbans forest of the Bay of Bengal, in the Ganges delta, where the bacterium *Vibrio cholera* had probably been mutating for millennia. The organism is found naturally in the environment in some coastal and brackish waters, where shellfish sometimes carry the infection.

Only in the early 1800s, however, when the British were opening up new trade routes in India and moving troops across the subcontinent, did cholera begin to move out of its home territory, first across India and eventually across the world in a series of huge pandemics. In August 1817, the British government received a report of a 'malignant disorder' in the Sundarbans, killing twenty to thirty people a day. Over the following few weeks, ten thousand people died. From there, the disease spread across the country and then fanned out eastwards and westwards to Nepal, Afghanistan, Iran, Iraq, Oman, Thailand, Burma, China and Japan.

This pandemic had hardly subsided when a second one began in 1826. Again the source was the Ganges Delta, and again the disease spread fast, revisiting old haunts but also travelling further, to the United States, Europe and Egypt. In Cairo and Alexandria alone, thirty-three thousand deaths were recorded in twenty-four hours.

By 1831, cholera was in Moscow, having decimated the great trading city of Astrakhan. When it reached St Petersburg, it had crossed the divide between Europe and Asia and was heading for Poland, Bulgaria, Latvia and Germany. The British were anxiously tracking its progress when the disease crossed the North Sea from Germany's Baltic coast to break out on the Sunderland quayside in the autumn of 1831. Over the following seventy years pandemics broke out in quick succession across the globe, affecting countries in every continent and killing countless millions.

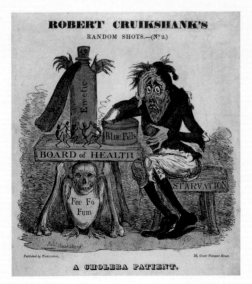

Left: Caricature of a cholera patient experimenting with remedies, c. 1832.

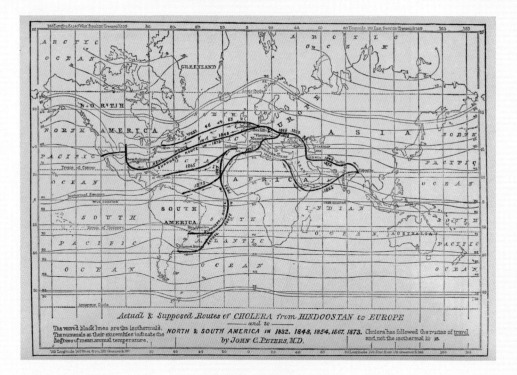

The waved black lines are the isothermals. The numerals at their extremities indicate the degrees of mean annual temperature.

Actual & Supposed Routes of CHOLERA from HINDOOSTAN to EUROPE
— and to —
NORTH & SOUTH AMERICA IN 1832, 1848, 1854, 1867, 1873. Cholera has followed the routes of travel and not the isothermal lines.
by JOHN C. PETERS, M.D.

Looking for answers

When cholera first appeared in Europe at the end of the 1820s, the developed world began to take notice. Doctors in Russia, France and Britain began studying the disease as a matter of urgency and the Russian government offered a prize of twenty-five thousand roubles (more than fifty thousand pounds today) for the best essay on the subject. But finding answers proved to be a difficult business.

With hindsight, it should have been obvious that cholera was contagious – that is, spread from person to person. It steadily followed the trade routes and appeared in new places only after the arrival of people from an infected area. Yet throughout most of the nineteenth century, there was huge debate about its mode of transmission. This was because of the way it killed large

Above: Map of actual and supposed routes of cholera from Hindoostan to Europe and the Americas in the nineteenth century.

numbers of people very fast and broke out seemingly at random, striking dozens or even hundreds overnight and then disappearing, only to reappear a few days later in some apparently unconnected place miles away. No other known disease behaved like this.

In the mid-nineteenth century, what was known as miasma – the foul smells given off by rotting organic material – was thought to be responsible for most epidemic diseases. Bad smells are, of course, a feature of poor hygiene, which does encourage disease. In 1846, the social reformer Edwin Chadwick told Parliament, 'All smell is disease'. The miasma theory

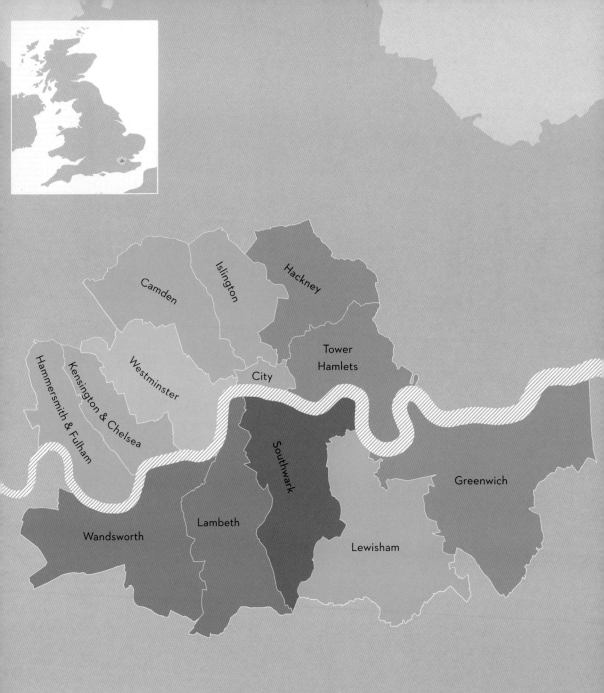

Hackney

Islington

Camden

Tower
Hamlets

Westminster

City

Hammersmith & Fulham

Kensington & Chelsea

Greenwich

Southwark

Lambeth

Lewisham

Wandsworth

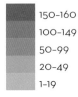

Cholera deaths recorded in London
in 1849 per 10,000 inhabitants

150–160

100–149

50–99

20–49

1–19

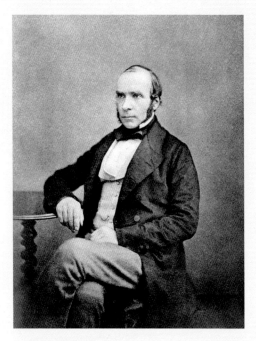

was just that, a theory, but some regarded it as a proven fact, and there was a debate between the 'contagionists' and the 'anti-contagionists'. One question was why, when a foul atmosphere polluted a wide area, did some people fall victim but others not.

Countless theories about cholera were put forward, including that the victims had an excess of carbon in their bodies. The suggestions about how to ward it off included sleeping with the bedroom door open, smoking tobacco or cannabis, avoiding vegetables, salads and pickles, and wearing shoes made of gutta percha, an early form of rubber.

The poor are usually hit disproportionately hard by disease because of insanitary living conditions, overwork and malnutrition. However, they are often blamed for bringing the illness on themselves through a dissolute lifestyle such as

from drinking alcohol. Cholera victims were no exception, although in London two particularly virulent outbreaks in 1848–9, one in a respectable middle-class street and the other among destitute children at a Dickensian 'child farm', exposed a flaw in that argument.

Then, in 1854, while Britain was in the throes of its third epidemic, a reclusive London physician made a massive breakthrough. He not only solved the mystery of cholera but also founded the science of epidemiology and pioneered the use of disease mapping, which is now a vital tool in investigating how diseases are spread. It was to be some years, however, before his thinking was accepted.

Infected drinking water

Dr John Snow's revolutionary theory posited that cholera's main route of transmission was through infected sewage finding its way into the water supply. He had noted that a seemingly random outbreak of cholera was always preceded by the arrival of someone from an infected district, and he suggested that transmission through drinking water would explain cholera's terrifying habit of striking large numbers of people at the same time.

South London had suffered badly in the 1848–9 outbreak. Homes there were

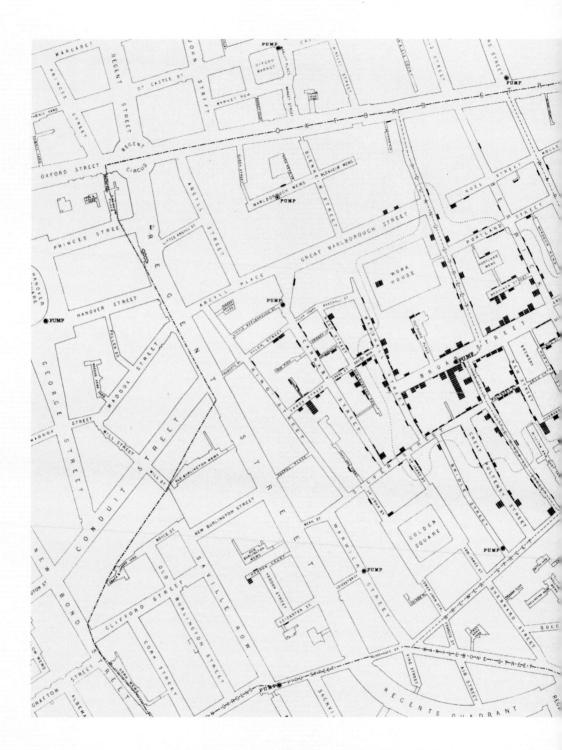

WATERBORNE

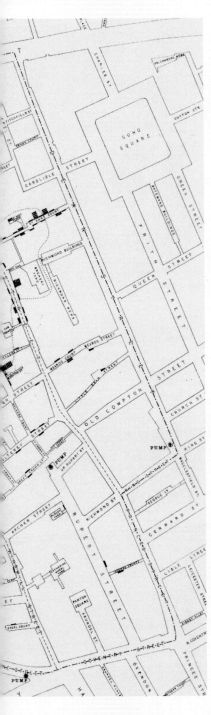

supplied with water by one of two companies, Lambeth or Southwark and Vauxhall. Both companies took their supplies from the Thames in London, next to a spot where the raw contents of the capital's sewers were discharged. The water was then pumped, unfiltered and untreated, into customers' homes. In 1852, however, Lambeth moved its works to rural Thames Ditton, well out of reach of the filth. Southwark and Vauxhall stayed where they were.

So, when the next epidemic broke out, Snow saw a way to prove his theory. He would compare the numbers of victims whose water was supplied by the two different companies during the 1848 epidemic, before Lambeth's clean-up, with the numbers of victims supplied by the two companies in 1854–5. If he was right, while customers of both companies were equally at risk in 1848, those with the clean Lambeth drinking water were now less likely to die.

He set off on what is now known as a 'shoe leather' investigation. Armed with a list of addresses where people had died, he began pounding the streets of south London, knocking on doors like a detective investigating a crime, asking the same question – which company supplied the household with water?

The results were clear. While in 1848 the customers of the two water companies were equally likely to die from cholera, in 1854 the mortality rate for those supplied by Southwark and Vauxhall was between eight and nine times higher than for those with the clean Lambeth water. This is now known as the Grand Experiment, and it is the first major study in the science of epidemiology that investigates how diseases are spread.

Street plan of death

As Snow was preparing to publish his research, his attention was caught by an event in London's West End. On the night of 31 August 1854, two hundred people living in a few lanes in Soho were simultaneously struck down with cholera. Ten days later the death toll was five hundred and rising.

Left: John Snow's iconic map of the 1854 cholera epidemic around Broad Street, Soho.

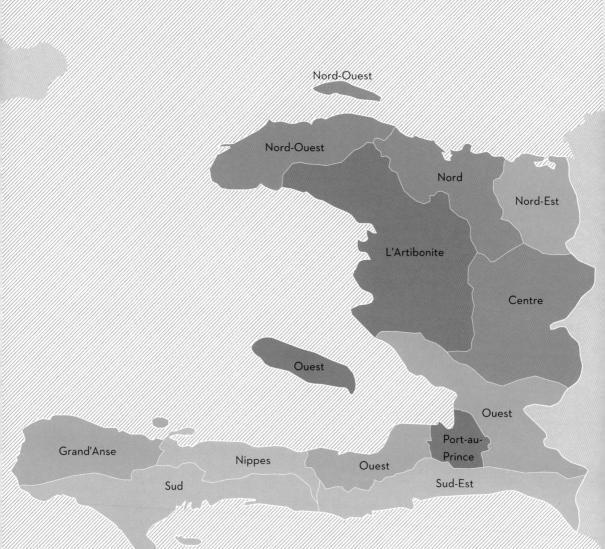

Nord-Ouest

Nord-Ouest

Nord

Nord-Est

L'Artibonite

Centre

Ouest

Ouest

Port-au-
Prince

Grand'Anse

Nippes

Ouest

Sud

Sud-Est

Reported cases of cholera in Haiti,
October 2010–January 2011

17,129–47,230

8,390–17,128

1,488–8,389

244–1,487

Snow took to the streets again, knocking on doors, this time collecting statistics on how many people had died and in which house. Then he went a step further, using what is now a key tool in tracking the spread of a disease. He marked on a street plan the buildings where people had died, a line for each death.

The death toll was by far the heaviest in one street, Broad Street, where the lines of deaths showed as large black blocks on most of the houses. And right at the centre of the outbreak stood the Broad Street pump. At every point where it was easier to go to another pump, the deaths tailed off or stopped altogether.

Snow also managed to explain a few cases that seemed at odds with his theory. The seventy men working at the Lion Brewery, right opposite the pump, all escaped unscathed. It turned out that one of the perks of the job was free beer; they never drank water. Equally, none of the 450 inmates of the local workhouse fell ill. The workhouse had its own water supply and never used the pump.

Modern outbreaks
During the second half of the nineteenth century, when people were provided with efficient sewers and clean drinking water, cholera largely disappeared in the developed world and the great global pandemics were consigned to history. However, the disease continues to be a threat when sanitary conditions are poor in countries where it is endemic, particularly when the infrastructure is damaged by natural disasters or war.

In 1961 a new, less deadly strain of the bacterium, known as El Tor, caused a pandemic that started in Indonesia and spread to Bangladesh, India, the Middle East, North Africa and by 1973 into Italy. A series of more deadly epidemics in the 1990s and 2000s killed tens of thousands of people, including those living in the Democratic Republic of Congo, Iraq, Zimbabwe and Nigeria.

In October 2010, cholera was confirmed in Haiti for the first time in a century, ten months after a catastrophic earthquake wrecked the country's fragile infrastructure and left hundreds of thousands of displaced people crammed into camps. That outbreak was the worst in recent history, with more than seven hundred thousand cases and nine thousand deaths. Since then, the number of cases has decreased steadily, but fatal outbreaks continue to emerge in the Caribbean, South America, the Middle East, the Indian subcontinent, Africa, the Far East, Yemen and Somalia. In the first half of 2017, there were 7,623 new cases and seventy deaths. Treatment is now available – antibiotics and rehydration therapy – but it has to be administered fast to be effective.

In 2017, the WHO published a strategy for reducing cholera deaths by 90 per cent by 2030. The key approach to controlling the disease is still decent sanitation. However, over the five years to 2018 more than fifteen million doses of an effective oral vaccine were given to people in areas where there was an outbreak or a humanitarian crisis or in 'hot spots' where cholera is highly endemic.

Meanwhile, the WHO classifies cholera not only as a global threat to public health but also as a key indicator of lack of social development. Cholera's secrets were finally revealed around 150 years ago, but the disease is still far from conquered.

Dysentery

||||||||||||||||

Causal agents:	Bacillary dysentery (shigellosis) the *Shigella* genus of bacteria
	Amoebic dysentery (amoebiasis)
	single-cell parasite, the *Entamoeba histolytica*
Transmission	Mainly contaminated food or water but also from one individual to another through infected faeces
Symptoms	Mainly watery diarrhoea flecked with blood, mucus or pus. Other symptoms include fever and chills, abdominal pain and weight loss.
Incidence	Shigellosis is responsible for an estimated 165 million cases of severe dysentery a year
Prevalence	Shigellosis and amoebiasis are endemic throughout the world
Prevention	Clean water, good sanitation and good hygiene practices, particularly hand-washing
Treatment	Antibiotics for shigellosis and antiparasitic drugs for amoebiasis. Rehydration to replace fluids and body salts lost through diarrhoea.
Global strategy	Provision of clean water, efficient sanitation and promotion of good hygiene practices

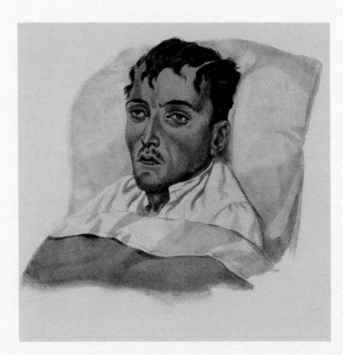

Illustration of a soldier suffering
from dysentery, from a German
publication on diseases, 1929.

The Crusaders of the Middle Ages were defeated 'not so much by the scimitars of the Saracens as by the hostile bacteria of dysentery and other epidemics', according to the nineteenth-century historian Charles Creighton. Whatever the truth of that claim, the disease decimated armies through the ages to the extent that it was often described as the 'fifth column' or 'the enemy within'.

Scourge of the battlefield

Dysentery ran through Napoleon's Grand Armée (Great Army), killing thousands and contributing to his defeat – along with typhus – in his ill-fated Russian Campaign of 1812. In the American Civil War of 1861–5, it was blamed for around forty-five thousand deaths in the Union Army and fifty thousand among the Confederates. Along with cholera, dysentery was rampant among soldiers in the Crimean War in 1853–6. When Florence Nightingale and her team arrived in 1854, among the horrors confronting them were two thousand dysentery patients in one hospital, left in squalor to recover or die.

The problem persisted well into the twentieth century and First World War in 1914–18, but reports linking dysentery epidemics with war go back as far as 480 BC and the Persian invasion of Greece. The exact death toll is unknown, but it is thought to be in the hundreds of thousands for a sickness that historians believe was either dysentery or plague.

No respecter of power or position, dysentery killed King John while he was fighting a campaign in eastern England in 1216 and struck down King Edward I while fighting the Scots in 1307. In 1422, during the Hundred Years' War, King Henry V died at the Château de Vincennes, outside Paris, apparently from the disease. Sir Francis Drake, Queen Elizabeth's Vice Admiral of the English fleet during the Spanish Armada, was another victim, succumbing in January 1596 while his ship was anchored off the coast of Portobelo in Panama. He had been keeping to his cabin and complaining of a 'scouring' or 'flux'. The 'bloody flux' was another name for dysentery.

In rural Ireland, dysentery seems to have been endemic for centuries. The Oxford scholar Anthony à Wood wrote that during Oliver Cromwell's siege of Drogheda in 1649, his brother Thomas, one of Cromwell's officers, 'ended his days of the country disease called the flux'. The leading seventeenth-century English physician Thomas Sydenham also wrote about 'the endemic dysentery of Ireland'. However, the history may go further back: Gerald of Wales, a priest and historian who accompanied the future King John on a military expedition to Ireland in 1185, referred to 'the Irish country disease'.

Cromwell's forces were struck again with what appeared to be dysentery during his attempts to colonise part of the Caribbean in 1655. Soon after the English fleet arrived at Santo Domingo in April, they were 'troubled with violent fluxes, hundreds having dropped down by the way, some sick, others dead'. Two weeks later another military dispatch reported: 'The rains increasing, our men weakening, even to death fluxing.' The enterprise had to be abandoned.

Disease of the vulnerable

Like most diseases, dysentery strikes the malnourished particularly hard. It is usually spread through contaminated food or water, often by flies, but it can also be passed from one individual to another through infected faeces, which is why handwashing is a vital part of prevention. It spreads fast where there is overcrowding and poor sanitation, which puts people living in confined and foul conditions such as refugee camps, institutions and army field camps at special risk. Sieges have been particularly dangerous, both for the besiegers and the besieged.

There are some terrible accounts of dysentery and other diseases on slave ships in the seventeenth and eighteenth centuries, where conditions were especially appalling. One report from Barbados in 1664 says:

> There has been a great mortality among the negroes, which the African Company's physician assures them is through a malignant distemper contracted, they think, through so many sick and decaying negroes being thronged together.

The slaves were in such a shocking state that most buyers rejected them. Philip Fusseires, 'a surgeon, to whom they sold 20 at a low rate' was said to have lost every one.

Another report, this time from Jamaica, tells how in 1672 a certain Captain James Tallers bought slaves off a ship that had just docked after three months at sea 'almost all starved and surfeycatted [surfeit had come to mean dysentery], he [the ship's captain] having fed them with little else but musty corn.' But even that was not enough to account for the men's condition, the writer thought, for he added: 'There must have been something extraordinary that so many died.'

As well as these specific outbreaks, epidemics also hit large sections of the general population. In the 1840s, at the height of the Irish potato famine, chronic dysentery, along with typhus, was reported to be widespread among the destitute, where it was known as starvation dysentery. Incidences also rose during the late nineteenth century when people began drinking more cow's milk. Untreated milk provides an excellent growth medium for the bacterium shigella, one of the main causes of dysentery.

Thomas Sydenham wrote about dysentery in London too, describing an outbreak in 1669 as the worst for ten years. From 1658 onwards, the disease features strongly in the London Bills of Mortality, which listed it in the causes of death under the term 'Griping of the guts'.

Disease of the intestines

The name 'dysentery' comes from the Greek language, meaning 'bad intestine'. It is a generic term for a group of diseases that can cause inflammation of the intestines and necrosis (death of the cells). The symptoms are diarrhoea containing blood or mucus. The World Health Organization (WHO) defines it as 'any diarrhoeal episode in which the loose or watery stools contain visible red blood'. It can take the form of a mild condition that clears up without treatment – or it can kill.

There are two main types. Bacillary dysentery, or shigellosis, caused by the *Shigella* genus of bacteria, is most common in Western countries. Amoebic dysentery, or amoebiasis – caused by a single-celled parasite, or amoeba, called *Entamoeba histolytica* – is found mainly in the tropics. Most people with amoebiasis have no symptoms but can develop bloody diarrhoea, fatigue, weight loss and occasional fever. The parasite can also spread to other organs, usually the liver, where it causes an abscess but it seldom kills. The exception is in people with the HIV virus, for whom the consequences can be severe.

Shigella dysenteriae type 1 is the most deadly of the bacteria and responsible for epidemics. The scientist Kiyoshi Shiga identified it in 1897 while investigating a large outbreak in Japan. Japan was hit by regular epidemics at the end of the nineteenth century: in a six-month period in 1897 more than ninety-one thousand people fell sick and twenty thousand died.

Spreading from Europe

Shigella was long thought to have originated in the tropics before then making its way into Europe. However, a 2016 study of more than than three hundred strains of bacteria across the world revealed that *Shigella dysenteriae* type 1, responsible for the large regional outbreaks and for the most severe disease, probably originated in Europe. At the end of the nineteenth century, it then broke out and swept round the globe, the researchers believed, carried by economic migrants into the United States and by colonialists into Africa, Asia and Central America.

Today, shigellosis is endemic throughout the world and is thought to be responsible for around 165 million cases of severe dysentery a year, killing more than a million people. The vast majority of cases are in developing countries and involve children under the age of five. Amoebiasis occurs worldwide too but is more common where sanitation is poor, particularly in the tropics.

Since the late 1960s shigellosis pandemics have hit sub-Saharan Africa, Central America and South and Southeast Asia, often where there is political upheaval or natural disaster. During the 1994

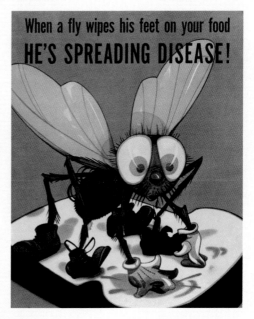

Above: American public health poster warning against flies and the spread of disease, 1944.

genocide in Rwanda, around twenty thousand refugees fleeing into Zaire died from dysentery in the first month.

Every year the United States sees about half a million cases of shigellosis. One outbreak in 2010 that struck 328 people in a small town near Chicago was traced back to two employees at the local Subway fast food restaurant.

One worrying emerging trend, now a feature of several infectious diseases, is drug resistance. The strain of shigella among Rwandan refugees proved able to withstand all of the then-usual antibiotics. Resistance to those drugs is now common and doctors have turned to alternatives. However, we are now beginning to see more new strains that are resistant to these drugs too. The pathogen is able to adapt with worrying speed.

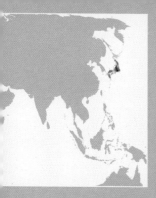

Recorded cases of dysentery
in Japan during 1897

9,000–10,000

5,000–8,999

2,000–4,999

1,000–1,999

500–999

1–499

Typhoid

⁞⁞⁞⁞⁞⁞⁞⁞⁞⁞⁞⁞

Causal agent	Bacterium *Salmonella Typhi*
Transmission	Contaminated food and water
Symptoms	Fever, fatigue, headache, nausea, abdominal pain, constipation or diarrhoea and sometimes a rash
Incidence and deaths	Estimated 11–20 million cases and 128,000–161,000 deaths a year worldwide
Prevalence	Global but mainly parts of Africa, the Americas, Southeast Asia and the Western Pacific
Prevention	Vaccination; provision of clean water, good sanitation and food hygiene
Treatment	Antibiotics but drug resistance is growing
Global strategy	US$85 million funding made available from 2019 for routine vaccination of children in countries where typhoid is endemic

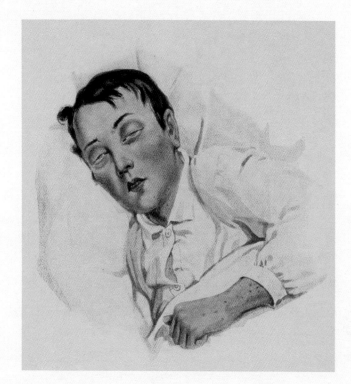

Illustration of a man suffering
with typhoid, from a German
publication on diseases, 1929.

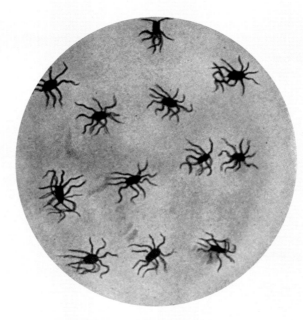

Above: *Illustration of the bacteria that cause typhoid fever.*

On the night of 28 April 1900, hundreds of British soldiers lay desperately sick, many of them dying. Their plight was made even worse by the conditions they were forced to endure: ten men crammed into tents meant for six, some with nothing but a blanket and a waterproof sheet between them and the hard ground. That night, 873 out of the 2,291 patients in the make-shift military hospitals in Bloemfontein during the Boer War were suffering from typhoid fever.

Estimates of the size of the Bloemfontein epidemic vary wildly, but it certainly killed thousands of men, some of whose chances of recovery were possibly reduced by a lack of care. Government commissioners looking into the medical arrangements heard some shocking testimony, and MP William Burdett-Coutts told them that the soldiers were 'dying like flies' from enteric fever.

An entwined history

Typhoid and paratyphoid, known jointly as enteric fever, are thought to have a long history in humans. The difficulty in tracking that history, however, is that the symptoms – fever, weakness, stomach pains, headache, constipation or diarrhoea and loss of appetite – are common to many other gastrointestinal diseases. A description of what appears to be typhoid is found in the writings of the fifth-century BC Greek physician Hippocrates, and a report of Emperor Caesar Augustus of Rome taking cold baths in order to treat a fever is thought to refer to the illness, but it is impossible to be sure.

In an outbreak in Jamestown, Virginia, in the seventeenth century, 6,500 out of 7,500 colonists died. During the American Civil War (1861–5), typhoid is thought to have killed around thirty thousand Confederate and thirty-five thousand Union troops. In the Spanish-American War of 1898, one-fifth of the US army were said to be affected, and six times more men died of the disease than those that died from wounds. Russia was also wracked by outbreaks in the 1920s.

Typhoid and paratyphoid are similar diseases, caused by different subspecies of the bacterium *Salmonella enterica*, but paratyphoid tends to be milder and has a lower mortality rate. The bacteria, which are found almost exclusively in humans, can be passed on in food or water contaminated with infected faeces or urine, or directly, for example, when a sick person with traces of faeces on their hands touches a healthy person. Flies can spread the disease if they land on faecal matter,

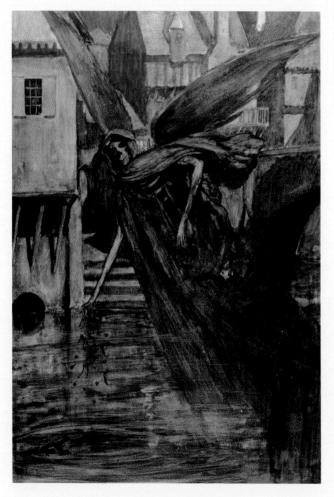

Left: *Watercolour depicting the angel of death dropping deadly substances into a river near a town; representing typhoid, c. 1912.*

and the infection can also be transferred, more rarely, on items such as handkerchiefs and towels. Enteric fevers are then, like cholera, strongly linked to the poor sanitation that prevails in slum housing, refugee camps and areas hit by natural disaster where the infrastructure – sewers and water supplies – has broken down.

More than 1,700 serotypes, or variations, of salmonella bacteria have been identified and most have both human and animal hosts. Human outbreaks have been traced to pet turtles, to drinking milk from infected cows and to eating infected eggs and poultry. Typhoid, though, is exclusively a human disease.

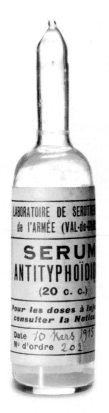

Above: *Ampoule of typhoid serum, 1915.*

Until the 1830s, typhoid and typhus were frequently confused, hence their similar names, although their causes and methods of transmission and some of their symptoms are different. A breakthrough came in 1850, when the British physician William Jenner distinguished the two diseases by systematically comparing their course, duration and symptoms.

Cleaning up the water

Another landmark came in 1873, when William Budd, another British physician, showed that the infection was mainly spread by water based on his observations over the previous forty years. The idea that a disease could be waterborne – first put forward by John Snow in relation to cholera in 1849 (see page 97) but only just gaining acceptance in the 1870s – revealed the importance of clean drinking water and good drains.

In the mid-nineteenth century, it was thought that typhoid, like other epidemic diseases, was caused by miasma, or foul smells, from rotting organic material. Budd argued, however, that typhoid did not arise spontaneously from filth but was contagious. In 1847, he studied a small typhoid outbreak in Clifton near Bristol and – again like John Snow investigating cholera in Soho in 1854 – he found that the key difference between those who fell sick and those who did not was that the victims had drunk from a particular well.

Revelations such as this prompted some key public health reforms in the industrialised world in the nineteenth century. In Britain, in particular, a series of major pieces of legislation led to a large drop in typhoid deaths, as well as the virtual disappearance of cholera. In 1862, the British medical journal *The Lancet*

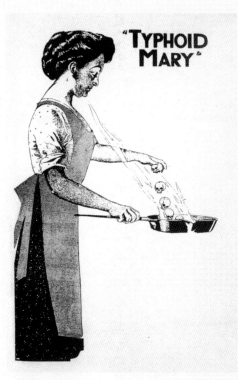

"TYPHOID MARY"

what his doctor William Jenner diagnosed as typhoid fever – the same doctor who had already helped to distinguish between typhoid and typhus. However, some modern-day experts now have their doubts. There is little doubt, though, about the sickness that nearly killed the then Prince of Wales, later King Edward VII. He was taken dangerously ill at Londesborough Lodge, Scarborough, exactly ten years after his father died. The event was said to have resulted in a new understanding of the importance of decent plumbing.

Even so, an investigation into the sanitary arrangements at Buckingham Palace in 1890 described the building as 'resting on a swamp of sewage through defective drainage'. It was made worse by a huge drain serving the nearby St George's Hospital that ran underneath the palace within a few feet of the basement, and which 'owing to faulty construction, was leaking in every direction'.

commented that the newly appointed medical officers of health had been so effective in cleaning up the inner cities that they had driven typhoid from working people's homes. However, the journal went on:

> the houses of the rich have not had the intelligent care and supervision which, by law, are given to the dwellings of the poor ... [and consequently] the middle classes of the metropolis are now suffering from fever – the fever of filth, of sewage gas and of tainted water.

In fact, the threat went to the very top of the social hierarchy. Queen Victoria's husband, Prince Albert, died at Windsor Castle in 1861, aged just forty-two, from

Typhoid Mary

In the United States, a clean-up of drinking water in the cities in the late nineteenth century saw the death rates from typhoid actually dip below those in the countryside. However, the continuing dangers were only too apparent as an extraordinary incident in New York State in 1906 was to show.

The wealthy banker Charles Warren hired a new cook, Mary Mallon, at his holiday home on Long Island. Over the space of a week, six out of eleven people

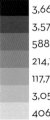

Figures for Typhoid fever
episodes in 2010

3,661,512
3,579,559
588,910
214,725
117,759
3,059
406

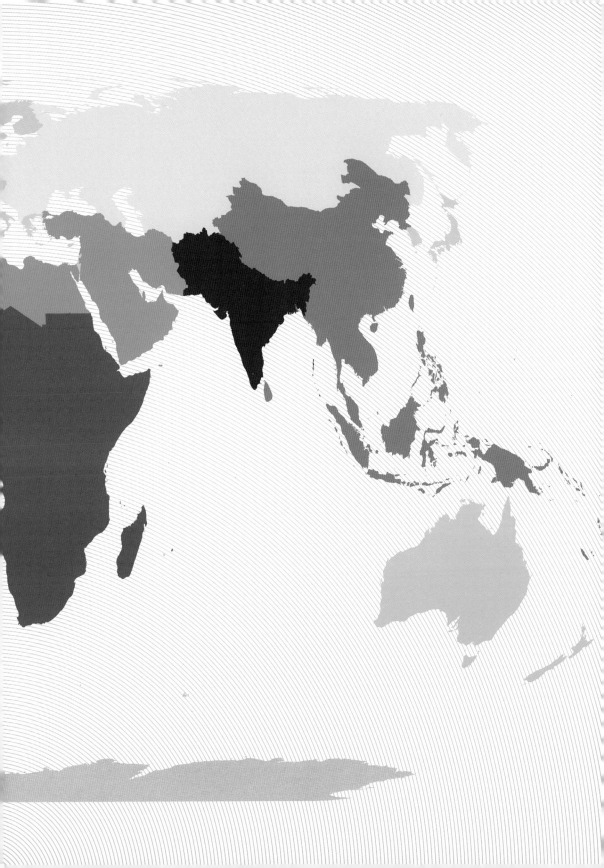

in the house went down with typhoid. A sanitary engineer, George Sober, was brought in to investigate. At first, he suspected that the local freshwater clams were the source of the trouble but then decided that Mallon, while healthy herself, was harbouring and spreading the bacteria. At that time, scientists were only just realising that some people could carry and spread the disease without falling sick themselves.

Sober began stalking a hostile Mallon, trying to obtain samples of her faeces, urine and blood. He was unsuccessful, but he did discover that seven out of eight families who had employed her had experienced cases of typhoid and some of the victims had died. That year, three thousand New Yorkers succumbed to the disease, an incident that has largely been blamed on Mallon.

The police who brought her in for testing were forced to overpower her. She was found positive for *S. typhi* and put into quarantine for three years. Mallon was released in 1910 on condition that she promised not to cook again. She began working as a laundress but went back to cooking because the wages were far higher. She managed to evade the authorities for five years, at one point taking a job in the kitchens of a Manhattan maternity hospital where, calling herself Mary Brown, she infected at least twenty-five people in three months, two of whom died. She was taken back into quarantine and remained there until her death in 1938.

A US public health official described the problem of carriers:

> The dirty man hanging on the car strap may be a typhoid carrier or it may be that the fashionably dressed woman who used it just before was infected with some loathsome disease. If these people were sick in bed we would avoid them. As it is, we cannot.

The story of 'Typhoid Mary', as Mallon was dubbed, has passed into folklore, but her case also became a cause celebre in a debate about the rights of the individual as against the rights of the state. Some also argued that she was treated particularly harshly because she was a poor Irish immigrant. 'I never had typhoid in my life and have always been healthy', she told a journalist. 'Why should I be banished like a leper and compelled to live in solitary confinement with only a dog for company?'

Mandatory immunisation

By 1900, when the Bloemfontein epidemic broke out, a typhoid vaccine was already available. Sir Arthur Conan Doyle, the creator of Sherlock Holmes and a retired doctor, went to South Africa to help care for the casualties. On his return, he argued for immunisation to be compulsory in the British army. At that time, most soldiers refused vaccination because of the side effects, even though the disease, like typhus, dysentery and syphilis – for which vaccines weren't, and still aren't, available – had for so many centuries been such a scourge in war zones. In the First World War, the British introduced mandatory immunisation and the troops stayed relatively free of typhoid.

Fast-forward to 2018, and typhoid is still a concern. An estimated eleven-to-twenty million people a year fall sick with the disease and between 128,000 and 161,000 die. While better living conditions and antibiotics have drastically reduced sickness and deaths in developed countries, in parts of Africa, the Americas,

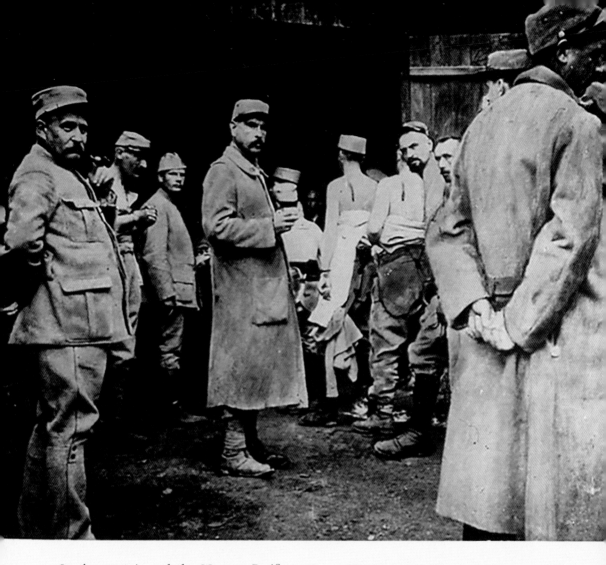

South-east Asia and the Western Pacific, typhoid remains a public health problem. In those regions, anyone without access to clean drinking water and decent sanitation is at risk, with children among the most vulnerable.

In 2017, experts advised the World Health Organization (WHO) that a new vaccine providing longer-lasting immunity should be given routinely to children more than six months old in countries where the disease is endemic. Soon afterwards, eighty-five million US dollars in funding

Above: Soldiers receiving the anti-typhoid vaccination during the First World War.

was made available for the vaccine, starting in 2019. Meanwhile, urbanisation and climate change 'have the potential to increase the global burden of typhoid', says the WHO, which also warns of the growing resistance to the antibiotics used to treat the disease.

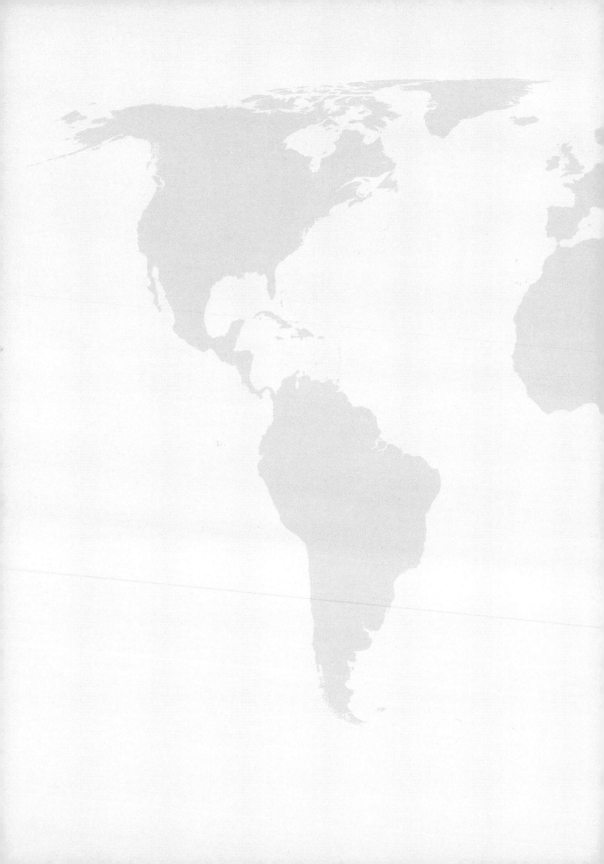

SECTION 3
INSECTS
& ANIMALS

Malaria

|||||||||||||

Causal agent	Species of the parasite plasmodium
Transmission	Bite from an infected female anopheline mosquito
Symptoms	Flu-like: malaise, fever, headache, sweats, chills, vomiting. Can include muscle pain and diarrhoea.
Incidence and deaths	216 million cases worldwide and 445,000 deaths in 2016
Prevalence	Found in more than 100 countries including large areas of Africa, Asia, Central and South America
Prevention	Drugs and environmental measures, including mass distribution of mosquito nets treated with insecticide
Treatment	Choice of drugs, depending on factors such as the type of parasite and the area where the infection was acquired
Global strategy	Prevention both environmental and drugs combined with fast diagnosis, treatment and surveillance. Goal of reducing incidence and mortality by at least 90 per cent by 2030.

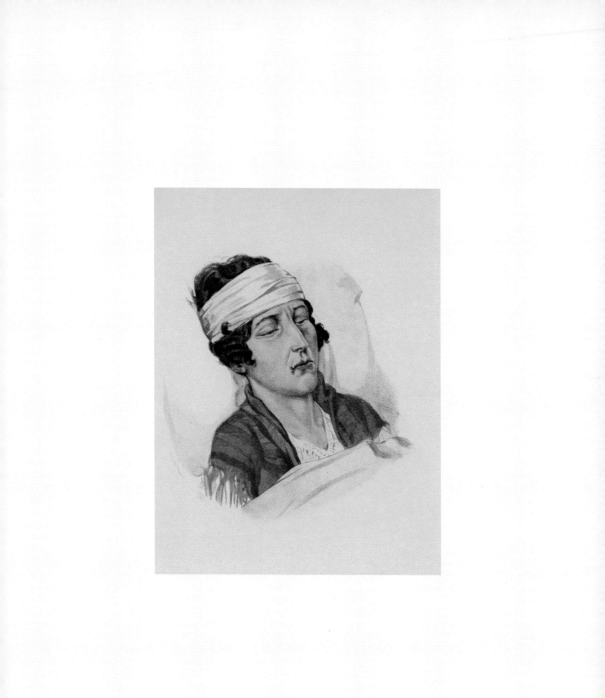

Illustration of a woman with
malaria, from a German publication
on diseases, 1929.

In 1740, the English politician Horace Walpole wrote to a friend to explain why he had left Rome: 'A horrid thing called mal'aria comes to Rome every summer and kills one.'

Centuries ago the links between the infection, marshy ground and a warm, damp climate were recognised. As with many epidemic diseases, though, the problem was thought to lie with foul smells – in this case the atmosphere of the swamps – hence the name 'mala aria', the Italian for 'bad air'. It was also known as swamp fever, ague and Roman fever,

the latter because, as Walpole noted, that city had a history of being plagued by the disease.

An age-old leading killer

Malaria ranks alongside tuberculosis and AIDS as one the world's leading killers. It is also one of the oldest-known infectious diseases, and scientific evidence suggests a long association between humans and the mosquito that spreads the disease. Because malaria leaves no trace on the bones, however, it is impossible to detect from skeletal remains.

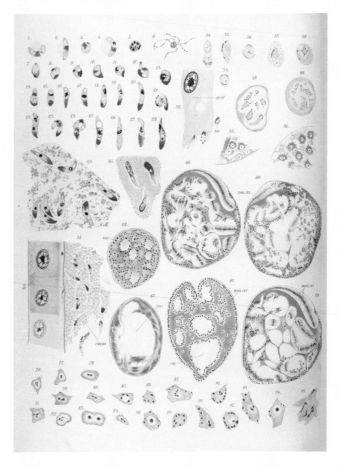

Right: *Illustration depicting cross-sections of parasites that cause malaria, 1901.*

The parasite responsible is thought to have begun as a single-cell plant like algae, for it appears to have been able to manufacture chlorophyll, which is essential for photosynthesis. At some point in its development, the parasite probably jumped species from monkeys to humans, and the disease that it causes possibly first appeared in South Asia before moving on to Africa and Europe and then the Americas.

In 2700 BC, several of malaria's characteristic symptoms were described in a Chinese medical text edited. In the fifth century BC, the Greek physician Hippocrates wrote what is thought to be an early description of the different cycles of symptoms caused by the different types of infection. He believed that the disease was caused by drinking stagnant water. The Sanskrit medical text *Sushruta Samhita*, whose origins probably date back to around 600 BC, also describes what might be malarial fever and says the condition was caused by insect bites.

During the Roman Empire malaria was common in Europe and around the Mediterranean basin. Initially, the disease was not as deadly as it was to become because the most lethal parasite involved, *Plasmodium falciparum*, was rare at the time. When two species of mosquito that carried the infection more effectively arrived in southern Europe from North Africa and Asia, however, this changed. In the final years of Rome's dominance, malaria was so deadly that some historians believe it helped to bring about the end of the empire, although plague is another contender here.

In medieval times and during the Renaissance malaria appears to have died down, but in the seventeenth and eigh-teenth centuries it was widespread in Europe once more, not only in the south but from time to time as far north as southern Scandinavia.

How malaria found its way to the Americas and the Caribbean is not understood but it may have arrived with Christopher Columbus and his crew at the end of the fifteenth century. At that time the infection was widespread in Europe and Africa and soon after the Europeans landed in the New World, there were reports of malaria spreading around the Caribbean. Not all parts of the New World provided a suitable environment or climate for the carrier mosquitoes, but by the nineteenth century the infection was widespread in the Mississippi Valley, the central valley of California and the coastal lowlands of northern South America.

Breakthroughs in scientific research

When the French chemist Louis Pasteur published his germ theory in the 1860s, scientists began to consider that an organism might be responsible for the disease. The first breakthrough came in 1880, when a French army surgeon, Alphonse Laveran, identified the parasite group that caused the infection in human beings. However, his findings were heavily contested as researchers were expecting bacteria to be responsible. Work then began on identifying the different types of parasite involved and the different species of mosquitoes that carried them.

In fact, there are four types of malarial infection caused by four species of a parasite called plasmodium. The marsh-land connection that the early physicians noted is, of course, where the mosquito is found. The most serious infection is from the *P. falciparum* parasite, which causes

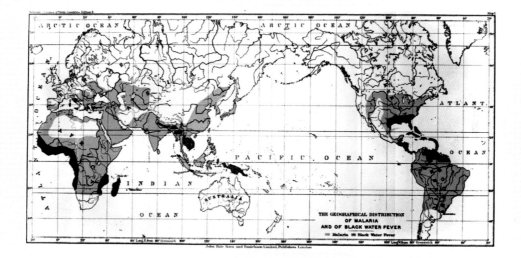

what is known as malignant tertian malarialternate bouts of chill, followed by high fever, sweating and prostration recur every forty-eight hours. The other three types are not usually life-threatening.

P. falciparum flourishes only in the tropics but another of the parasites, *P. vivax*, tolerates lower temperatures and has been found in Britain and southern Canada. It has been suggested that Europeans brought *P. vivax* to the New World, while African slaves introduced the *P. falciparum* parasite. In the Caribbean, the slaves' apparent inborn immunity that helped them survive *P. falciparum* unfortunately made them even more valuable as slaves. When the Europeans, with no immunity, came into contact with *P. falciparum* for the first time, the effects were devastating and are said to have helped dig what was known as the White Man's Grave in parts of Africa.

The big advance in understanding the disease came in 1897 when Ronald Ross of the British Indian Army Medical Corps showed that an infected person could pass the malaria parasite to a mosquito. He went on to show that the mosquitoes, in turn, could transmit the parasite to birds and from one bird to another, so demonstrating how the infection was spread. Ross received the Nobel Prize in Physiology or Medicine in 1902.

The only known carrier of human malaria is an infected female anopheline mosquito, of which some sixty different species exist in various parts of the world. In 1898 an Italian team described the full life cycle of the parasite in humans.

Environmental conditions

While the laboratory work on the micro-biology of malarial spread was underway, some research on the ground looked at the environmental factors involved. In the mid-nineteenth century, a deadly epidemic broke out on two islands in the Indian Ocean but not on three other islands nearby. Researchers suggested that the

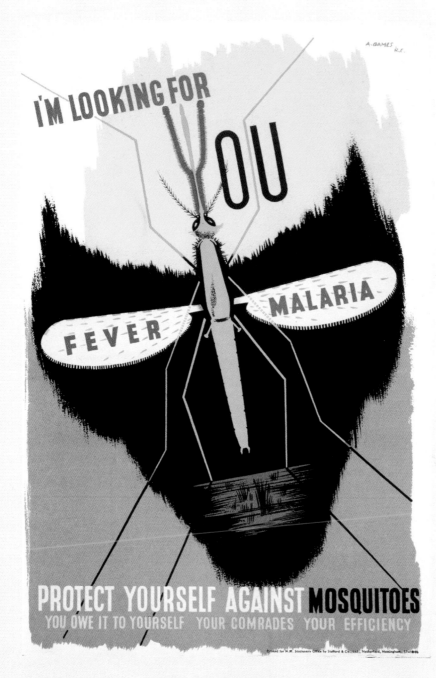

Above: *Malaria poster from 1941, warning against mosquitoes, with the wings of the insect forming the eye sockets of a skull.*

massive deforestation, carried out in order to cultivate sugar cane, combined with natural phenomenon such as cyclones, had created the perfect conditions for malaria mosquitoes from Africa to flourish. The disease was eventually brought under control, but there is a continuing risk of its reintroduction.

In the twentieth century, understanding the parasite's life cycle was a key to improving control, for example, through the use of insecticides. By the early 1950s countries such as Italy, the United States and Romania introduced eradication programmes, but across the world malaria still posed a massive threat. One official estimate put the global figures at three hundred million cases a year and more than three million deaths.

The construction of the Panama Canal, at the beginning of the twentieth century, was only made possible when malaria and yellow fever were brought under some control. The Isthmus of Panama is an ideal environment for mosquitoes: a constant high temperature; a nine-month rainy season and a tropical jungle. When work on the canal began, an estimated one-sixth of the population of the city of Colon, near the entrance to the canal, was suffering from malaria in any given week.

In 1901, the United States helped the Cuban city of Havana control another mosquito-borne disease, yellow fever, by quarantining new arrivals, mosquito-proofing buildings and draining the swamps. The measures were successful and had the additional benefit of greatly reducing the incidence of malaria. Based

Below: The World Health Organization Interim Committee on malaria, 1947.

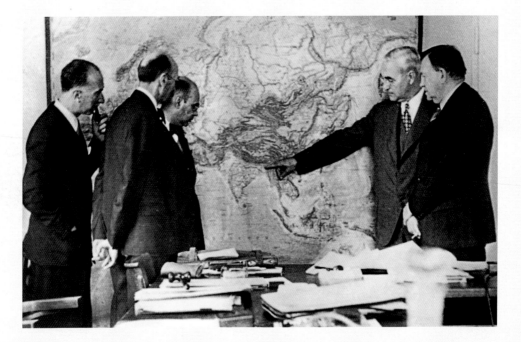

on that experience, sanitation experts drew up anti-malaria plans for the Panama Canal zone and the nearby cities.

During 1906, out of around 26,000 people working on the canal, more than 21,000 were hospitalised with malaria. By 1912, however, only 5,600 out of 50,000 went to hospital. And over the three years to the end of 1909, death rates also dropped dramatically, both among the workers and in the total population. But the disease remained a challenge throughout the project.

In the 1940s, DDT (dichlorodiphenyl-trichloroethane), was introduced, the first modern synthetic insecticide. It proved highly effective in combatting malaria, yellow fever, typhus and the other insect-borne diseases and was also widely used in farming and in homes and gardens. But then in the 1960s, concerns started to be raised about the damage it was doing to the environment as well as the risk it posed to human health.

In 2004, the Stockholm Convention on Persistent Organic Pollutants came into force, a global treaty banning DDT except for malaria control. In 2006, the World Health Organization (WHO) declared its support for the indoor use of DDT in African countries where malaria remained a major health problem, saying that the benefits outweighed the risks.

The Challenge to Eradicate

In 1955, the WHO had announced plans to eradicate malaria across the globe but the programme ended in 1969, widely considered a failure. By 2015, the goal had been revised to reducing incidence and mortality rates by at least 90 per cent by 2030. The strategy consists of prevention – both environmental and drugs – fast diagnosis, treatment and surveillance. In 2014–16, 582 million mosquito nets treated with insecticide were distributed, 505 million of them in sub-Saharan Africa.

In 2016, forty-four countries reported fewer than ten thousand cases, up from thirty-seven countries in 2010, while Kyrgyzstan and Sri Lanka were certified as malaria free and twenty-one countries identified as capable of eliminating the disease by 2020.

At the same time, however, after what the WHO called 'an unprecedented period of success in controlling malaria', by 2017 progress had stalled. In 2016, there were 216 million cases worldwide, an increase of about five million over the previous year, and 445,000 deaths. Africa accounted for 91 per cent of all deaths, the vast majority in sub-Saharan countries.

The WHO blamed inadequate funding, saying that to reach the first milestone – a reduction of at least 40 per cent in incidence and mortality compared with 2015 – investment needed to more than double. There was also the need for constant vigilance. After malaria cases had been reduced to zero in a particular area or country, preventing re-establishment then became a key concern. Scientists are also warning that climate change and global warming are likely to see the appearance or reappearance of the malaria-carrying mosquito in areas where it is currently not seen.

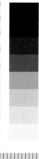

Number of malaria cases in
2016 (in 1,000)

100,001 to 250,000

50,001–100,000

5,001–50,000

1,001–5,000

501–1,000

51–500

5–50

0–4

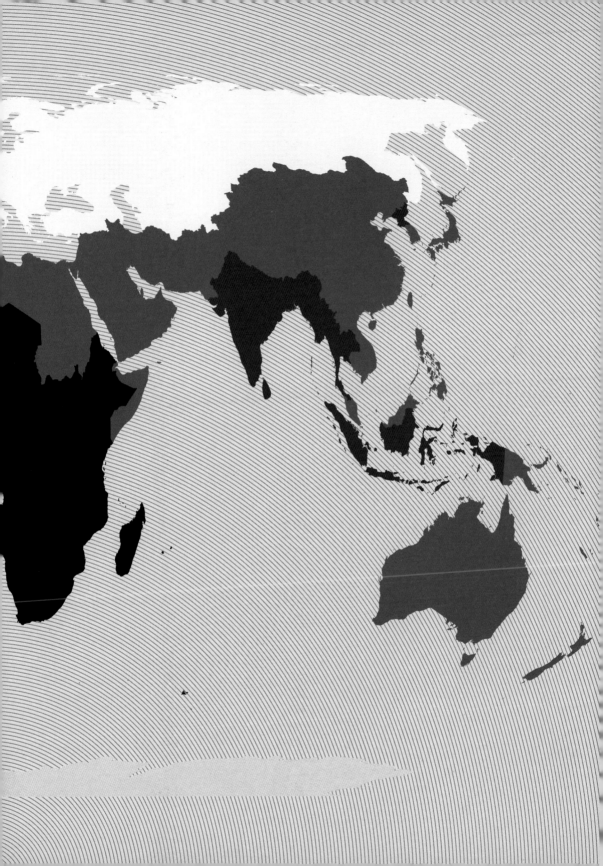

Number of malaria deaths in 2016

30,001–450,000

10,001–30,000

5,001–10,000

1,001–5,000

1–1,000

0

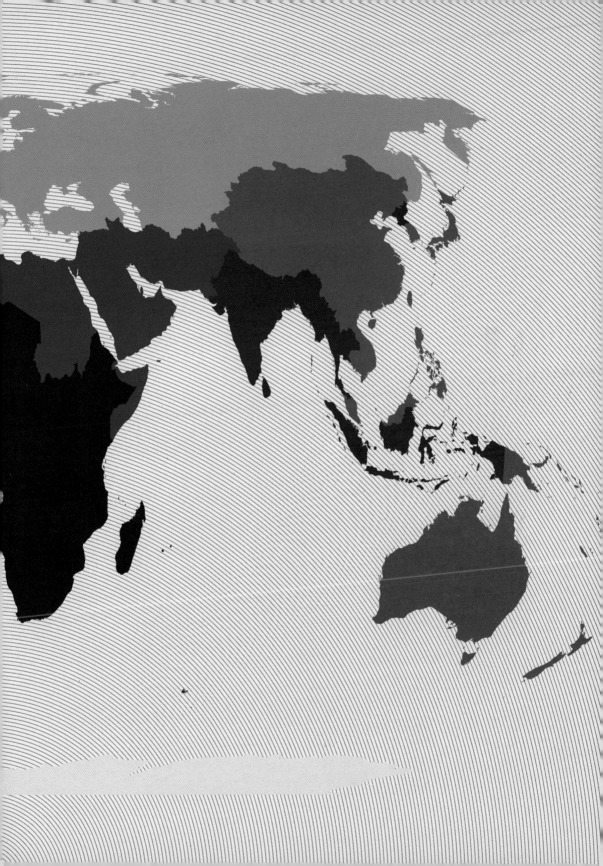

Plague

||||||||||||||||

Causal agent	Bacterium *Yersinia pestis*
Transmission	From rodents to humans by flea bite. Also person to person through respiratory route or direct contact with infected tissue.
Symptoms	Fever, chills, head and body aches, and weakness, vomiting and nausea. In bubonic plague – the most common type – painful swollen lymph nodes that can turn into pus-filled open sores.
Incidence and deaths	3,248 cases and 584 deaths worldwide in 2010–15. Case-fatality ratio of 30 to 60 per cent for bubonic plague. Pneumonic, second most common type, is invariably fatal if untreated.
Prevalence	Endemic in many rural areas in the Americas, Africa and Asia but mostly in the Democratic Republic of the Congo, Madagascar and Peru
Prevention	Destruction of rodent habitats and use of insecticides where the disease is endemic
Treatment	Antiobiotics along with oxygen therapy and intravenous fluids
Global strategy	Surveillance of at-risk areas and fast response to contain outbreaks

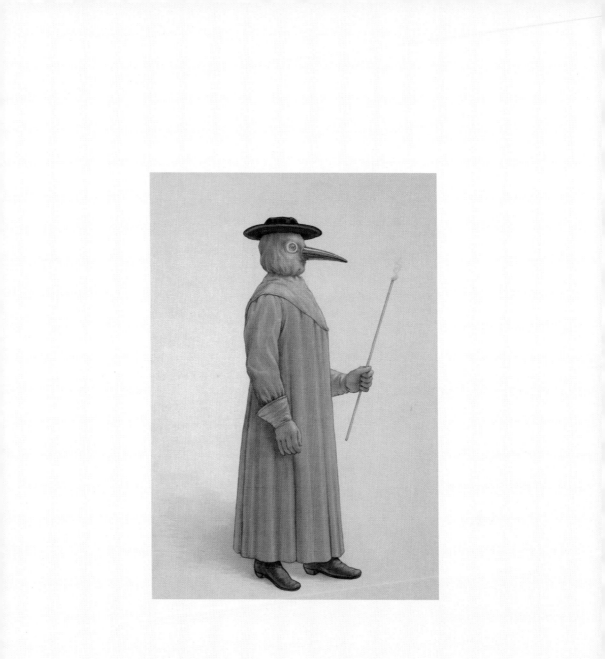

A physician wearing a seventeenth-century
plague-preventive costume.

For centuries, plague has caused havoc across continents, changing economies, political structures and social hierarchies. Its name, from the Latin for 'wound' or 'strike', still has the power to terrorise and is used to describe all manner of disasters, including the ten plagues in the Hebrew Bible.

Plague goes back a long way: researchers announced in 2017 they found plague in human remains in Russia and Croatia dating back to the late Stone Age. Some historians suggest that the deadly 'plague' that hit Rome in AD 165 helped to bring about the fall of the Roman Empire, although it's not certain that this was bubonic plague or another epidemic disease such as smallpox. Regardless, plague is responsible for three major pandemics.

The Justinian Plague

The first recorded pandemic – in fact, the first major outbreak of any disease to be reported with much reliability – is known as the Justinian Plague, named after the then Byzantine emperor. It began in AD 541 in Constantinople (modern-day Istanbul), before spreading east into Persia and west into southern Europe, eventually killing an estimated 33 to 40 per cent of the world's population.

While the plague's progress after Constantinople is mapped, it is still unclear how the disease reached the city. The Byzantine historian Procopius, who witnessed the devastation, claimed plague came from Egypt, following the trade routes. More recent theories suggest it originated in sub-Saharan African, possibly Kenya, Uganda, and/or Zaire, before either moving into Egypt or taking a different route to the Byzantine capital. Other experts believe the source was from the region spanning what is now Russia and China, now generally agreed to be the source for the Black Death some eight hundred years later.

Typically, when winter arrived in Constantinople, plague petered out, only to erupt again across the Byzantine Empire the following spring. The epidemics then continued sporadically until the eighth century.

The disease is caused by the bacterium *Yersinia pestis*, which is usually spread from rodents to humans by the bite of an infected flea, but it can also be spread by either inhaling droplets when a victim coughs or sneezes or by direct contact with

Below: Lithograph entitled The Dance of Death, *c. 1831.*

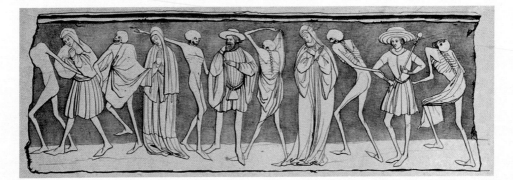

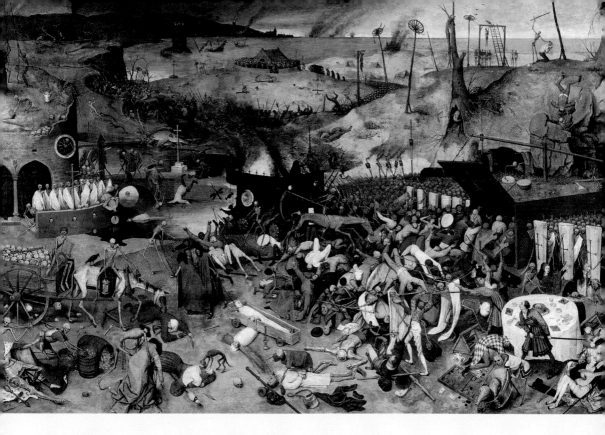

infected tissue. However, in one study in early 2018, researchers cast doubt on the role of the rat in the pandemic known as the Black Death, claiming it did not account for the disease's rapid spread across the world. They reported that plague was more likely to have been spread by fleas and lice living on human bodies and clothing.

There are two main forms of infection: bubonic and pneumonic. Bubonic plague, concentrated in the lymph nodes, is more common. Pneumonic plague, centred in the lungs, is more deadly but less easily caught and makes up only a small number of cases. A third variety, septicaemic plague, occurs when the bacteria enter the bloodstream.

The Black Death
Bubonic plague's painful swollen lumps, the notorious black 'buboes' in the neck,

Above: The Triumph of Death, c. *1562 by Peter Brueghel the Elder.*

armpits and groin, are infamous. In the fourteenth century, the Welsh poet Jeuan Gethin wrote: 'Woe is me of the shilling in the arm-pit; it is seething, terrible, wherever it may come, a head that gives pain and causes a loud cry, a burden carried under the arms.'

The Black Death is often described as the worst pandemic in history, killing an estimated 60 per cent of Europe's eighty million population and and between seventy-five million to two hundred million people across the world. It was long thought to have originated in China but another theory is that it began in the vast Euro-Asian Great Steppe region. Here, a plague reservoir – an area where the

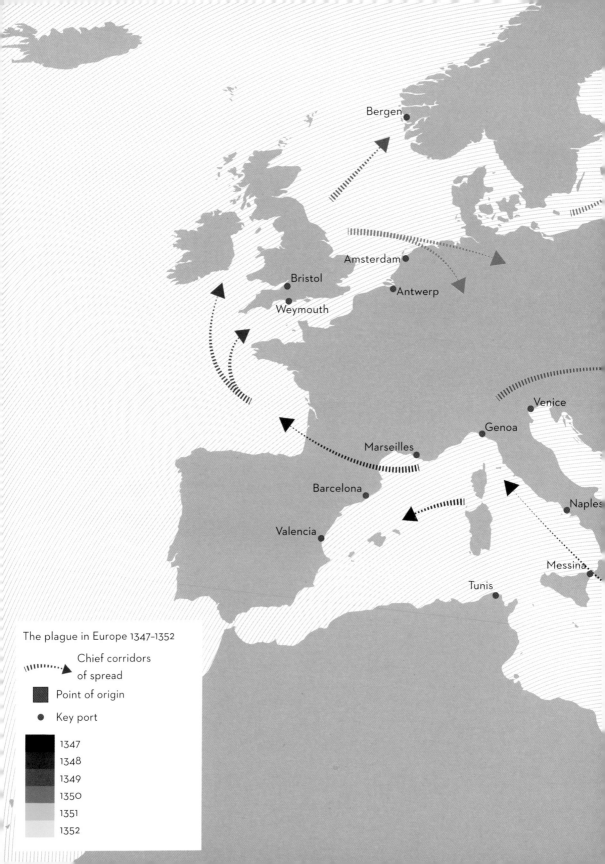

The plague in Europe 1347–1352

Chief corridors
of spread

Point of origin

Key port

1347
1348
1349
1350
1351
1352

Bergen

Bristol
Weymouth

Amsterdam
Antwerp

Venice
Genoa
Naples
Messina

Marseilles
Barcelona
Valencia
Tunis

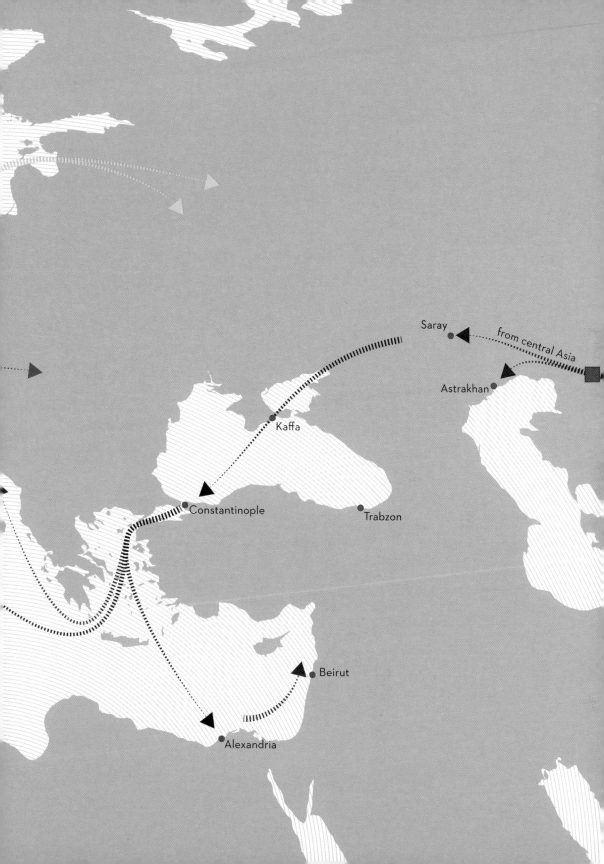

Saray

from central Asia

Kaffa

Astrakhan

Constantinople

Trabzon

Beirut

Alexandria

bacterium is rife among densely packed colonies of wild rats – stretches from the northwestern shores of the Caspian Sea into southern Russia.

The first cases have been traced to a Mongol attack on an Italian trading station in the Crimea in 1346. Plague broke out among the Mongols and spread into the town. When the Italian merchants fled home, their ships docked at various ports along the way, and they took the infected rats with them.

Florence and Siena were badly hit. The poet Petrarch said those who had not witnessed the unfolding tragedy would never believe the scale of the devastation. Instead they would, he said, 'look upon our testimony as a fable'. A shoemaker from Sienna, Agnolo di Tura, who lost five of his children, wrote:

> It is impossible for the human tongue to recount the awful truth ... None could be found to bury the dead for money or friendship. Members of a household brought their dead to a ditch as best they could, without priest, without divine offices.

This picture of the bodies piling up faster than the authorities could bury them is now indelibly linked with plague.

Following the shipping trade routes

The unprecedented spread of the Black Death has been linked to the great expansion in trade then taking place across Europe. The latest ships could carry larger cargoes over longer distances: the new routes now connected the Italian ports of Venice and Genoa with Constantinople and the Crimea, Alexandria and Tunis, and London and Bruges. And from London and Bruges, the sea link continued on to the Nordic countries and the Baltic.

The Italian vessels from the Crimea arrived in Constantinople in May 1347 and the epidemic broke out there in early July. More ships carried the disease from Constantinople to Alexandria, from where it spread into North Africa, across the Middle East and around the Mediterranean, reaching Marseilles in September. From Marseilles, it moved northwards, up the Rhône Valley to Lyons and southwest to Spain. The Italian merchants' ships meanwhile sailed on to Genoa, Venice and Pisa.

Soon the disease was attacking Spain from two separate fronts, while in France it moved west towards Brittany, southeast towards Paris and north to Holland and Belgium. Meanwhile, another plague ship had docked at Rouen in Normandy.

Plague arrived in England in June 1347 from southwest France at what is now Weymouth on the Dorset coast. The country was then attacked via its seaports on several fronts, as on mainland Europe: at Bristol in the southwest, Colchester and Harwich in the east and Grimsby in the north. London was hit in August. Soon the infection was rife across the entire country. Scotland, Wales and Ireland all followed.

Norway, Denmark, Sweden, Germany, Austria, Switzerland and Poland succumbed either around the same time or soon after. Russia was struck towards the end of 1351. Iceland and Finland, with tiny populations and few contacts with the outside world, are the only regions in Europe that the experts are fairly confident escaped.

But while populations and travel were increasing across Europe, helping to spread infections, there was little understanding of how diseases were transmitted

The Great Plague of London

The first recorded cases of the 'Great Plague of London' were diagnosed early in 1665 when two people died in Drury Lane in Westminster, outside the city walls. Dr Nathaniel Hodges, who stayed in London treating patients throughout the disaster, claimed that the tragedy could have been prevented if only the authorities had acted faster. Hodges wrote:

> Some timorous neighbours ... removed into the City of London, who unfortunately carried along with them the pestilential taint; whereby that disease, which was before in its Infancy ... suddenly got strength, and spread abroad its fatal poisons; and merely for want of confining the persons first seized with it, the whole city was in a little time irrecoverably infected.

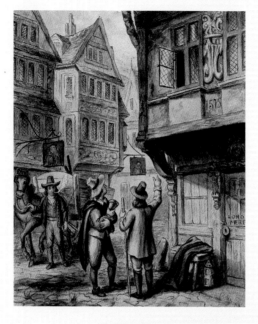

Above: *A cart for transporting the dead in London during the Great Plague, 1665.*

and, therefore, no effective attempts to prevent them. Epidemics in general, and plague in particular, were seen as God's punishment for sin. The response therefore was either penitence or fatalism.

The Black Death finally petered out in 1453 although the disease continued to recur here and there in small sporadic outbreaks. In England, it persisted into the early fifteenth century. In 1563, more twenty thousand people died in London, between one-quarter and one-third of the city's population. Experts have argued that the massive toll taken by the Black Death in the late Middle Ages had an upside: the resulting labour shortage forced through major social reforms as well as sped up advances in technology.

In the hot summer, the death toll climbed relentlessly until by September it had reached 7,165 a week. Most of the wealthy and powerful fled, including the Royal Court, lawyers and Parliament. The Lord Mayor though stayed to enforce the emergency regulations aimed at containing the spread. Victims were locked into their houses and provided with food, while paid 'searchers' looked for dead bodies and trundled them out by the cartload at night to be buried in pits outside the City walls. The poor, fleeing on foot into the surrounding countryside, were attacked by locals and chased away. The precautions failed to protect London from devastation but the epidemic was largely contained within the City.

One exception that has passed into legend in Britain is that of the village of Eyam in Derbyshire. Eyam was struck in September, it is claimed through a bale of cloth from London that was infested with

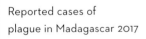

Reported cases of
plague in Madagascar 2017

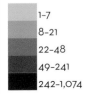

1–7
8–21
22–48
49–241
242–1,074

fleas. When plague began spreading, the vicar persuaded the villagers to put themselves into quarantine. Of around 350 villagers, 259 were said to have died. It is easy to see why this story has caught the public imagination but modern historians question some aspects, claiming that, at most, 50 per cent of the villagers died and that the quarantine was not unique to Eyam.

Typically, as the autumn temperatures dropped, the plague began to wane. In mid-October the diarist Samuel Pepys wrote: 'But Lord, how empty the streets are, and melancholy, so many poor sick people in the streets, full of sores ... but there are great hopes of a great decrease this week. God send it.' Pepys' hopes were realised. The Great Plague of London was coming to an end. The official death toll was put at 68,596, but the true number is thought to be more than one hundred thousand.

The Modern Plague

The third and last pandemic, known as the Modern Plague, began in China in the 1860s and had reached Hong Kong by 1894. Over the next twenty years, in what was then a familiar pattern, it spread to port cities around the world, eventually causing an estimated ten to twelve million deaths. More recent epidemics have broken out in India in the first half of the twentieth century, and in Vietnam during the war in the 1960s and 1970s. Plague is now commonly found in sub-Saharan Africa and Madagascar, which areas now

account for more than 95 per cent of reported cases.

The Modern Plague though coincided with huge scientific advances in our understanding of infectious disease. Building on Louis Pasteur's germ theory, researchers in the late nineteenth and early twentieth centuries were identifying the various bacteria responsible for different diseases. In 1894, as the Modern Plague arrived in Hong Kong, the French bacteriologist Alexandre Yersin identified the organism that causes plague and explained its mode of transmission.

Soon after, rat-associated plague was brought under control in most urban areas, but in the Americas, Africa and Asia the infection spread easily to local populations of ground squirrels and other small mammals. These new species of carriers have allowed the disease to become endemic in many rural areas, including the western United States. As of October 2017, however, plague was most endemic in the Democratic Republic of the Congo, Madagascar and Peru.

Because plague spreads so fast and has such a high casualty rate, the bacterium *Yersinia pestis* has been used as a weapon in crude forms of biological warfare for centuries, with corpses being catapulted over city walls and infected fleas dropped from planes. In recent times, the bacterium has been identified as a security threat because of its possible use by terrorists. An expert panel in the United States has warned about the deadly potential of 'an aerosolized plague weapon'.

Typhus

||||||||||||||||

Causal agent	The *Rickettsia prowazekii*, a type of bacteria
Transmission	By the human body louse, *Pediculus humanus corporis*
Symptoms	Headache, chill, prostration, high fever, coughing and severe muscle pain, followed by a dark spot on the upper trunk, spreading to the entire body excepting, usually, the face, palms and soles of the feet
Incidence	Since the Second World War most reported outbreaks have been in Burundi, Ethiopia and Rwanda. 20,000 cases in Burundi in 1997
Prevalence	Colder regions of Central and Eastern Africa, central and South America, and Asia, where there is overcrowding and poor hygiene, such as in prisons and refugee camps
Prevention	General cleanliness and use of insecticides in cases of louse infestation
Treatment	One dose of an antibiotic

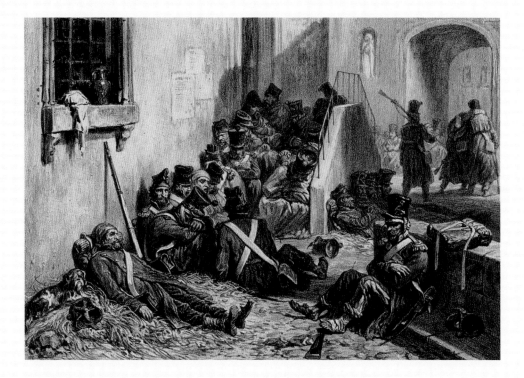

*Nineteenth-century lithograph of soldiers
suffering from typhus, lying in the
streets of Mainz, Germany.*

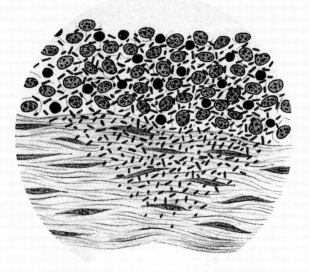

Above: *Depictions of typhus bacillus-infected intestine*

'The history of typhus ... is the history of human misery.' So wrote the nineteenth-century epidemiologist August Hirsch. Hirsch singled out typhus because back through the centuries it targeted those who were already in the most wretched conditions: rotting in prisons, crammed into foul slums, starving in famines and fighting on battlefields. As a result, it has been known as jail fever, camp fever and war fever. Because of its association with those who were sometimes described as 'the great unwashed', the victims themselves have sometimes been blamed.

Looking back to earlier times of war and famine, it can be hard to separate the typhus deaths from those caused by dysentery or starvation as the three often go hand in hand. The potato famines in Ireland in the eighteenth

and nineteenth centuries are a perfect example of this.

Epidemic typhus is caused by the organism *Rickettsia prowazekii*, one of a group responsible for a range of diseases, including Rocky Mountain spotted fever, rickettsialpox, African tick bite fever and Australian tick typhus. Rickettsiae are tiny bacteria, of a type known as intracellular gram-negative bacteria.

R. prowazekii is spread by the human body louse, *Pediculus humanus corporis*, which lives in clothing and becomes infected by feeding on the blood of someone with typhus fever. Infected lice then excrete rickettsiae onto the skin while feeding on a second host, who becomes infected by rubbing the faecal matter or crushed lice into the bite wound. Head lice and pubic lice have no role to play. The lice spread fast in crowded insanitary conditions, particularly in cold and wet weather when people wear more clothing and use more blankets.

Was the first epidemic typhus?

Historians believe that typhus has a long history although its origins are unclear. Some think that the so-called Plague of Athens in 430 BC – the first documented major epidemic, which broke out during the Peloponnesian War – was typhus. The death toll has been put at between seventy-five thousand and one hundred thousand, about 25 per cent of the city's population, but even giving an estimate of these numbers is difficult.

The Greek historian Thucydides survived the Athens epidemic and went on to write a colourful account of the symptoms. They began, he said, with 'violent heats' in the head, inflammation of the eyes, and 'the inward parts, such as the throat or tongue, becoming bloody and emitting an unnatural and fetid breath'. Sneezing and coughing followed, then diarrhoea, vomiting and violent spasms. Next came pustules and ulcers all over the body and a burning, unquenchable thirst. Most people died around the seventh or eighth day. This wide-ranging list puts other diseases in the frame, however, including smallpox, typhoid, bubonic plague and even ebola.

A regular in Europe's wars and prisons

Not until the fifteenth century do the records become more reliable, largely from European wars. Typhus appears to have established itself on the continent in 1489–90 at the end of Spain's eight hundred-year-old fight to reclaim the Iberian Peninsula from the Moors. The Spanish lost thousands of men to typhus at the battle of Granada. Then began a long series of epidemics that would strike armies in some of the most famous military campaigns through the coming centuries, including the Ottoman Wars, the Thirty Years' War, the Baltic Wars and the English Civil War. In 1812, the disease was said to have played as great a part in Napoleon's retreat from Moscow as did the Russian army and the Russian winter.

Typhus was also a regular visitor to English prisons and courtrooms for hundreds of years. So many prisoners died in filthy overcrowded jails that – at a time when executions were commonplace – typhus was said to kill more criminals than the hangman. An epidemic at the Oxford summer assizes in 1577 – afterwards known as the Black Assizes – killed more than three hundred people, including Sir Robert Bell, the Lord Chief Baron of the Exchequer. During the Lent assizes in the southwest of England in 1730, the High Sheriff, the judge, the serjeant at law and the court crier all died.

In 1737, the courtroom at London's Old Bailey was enclosed and a passage built to link the building to Newgate Prison next door. But what were intended as improvements only served to increase the risk of infection, and in 1750 a typhus epidemic killed sixty people, mainly prisoners but also the Lord Mayor and two judges. An inquiry blamed the appalling conditions caused by, the investigators said, 'the horrid neglect of gaolers'. Because stuffy air and bad smells were thought to cause disease, judges began to bring herbs and flowers into the court to mask the stench, and the practice is commemorated in a ceremony today.

Irish fever

During the eighteenth and nineteenth centuries, Ireland was plagued by outbreaks, all of them linked to failures of the potato crop, the food staple of the poor. In 1847, in what was known as the Great Famine, so many sick and starving Irish immigrants arrived in Liverpool that the city ran out of hospital beds. Typhus patients were nursed in temporary wards set up in dockside warehouses, known as fever sheds.

At one point, sixty thousand people in Liverpool were sick, the vast majority of them Irish, so typhus became known as Irish fever. Some of the locals said that the Irish only had themselves to blame, as the disease, they claimed, was the result of drunkenness and dissolute living.

In Canada the story was the same. The typhus epidemic of 1847 killed more than twenty thousand, mainly Irish immigrants who had caught the disease on one of the coffin ships, so-called because they were so crowded and unseaworthy.

New World typhus

Whether or not the disease was in the New World before Columbus arrived is not known, but it seems to have crossed the Atlantic at some point during the second half of the sixteenth century and is a contender for the disease known as cocoliztli, which killed around two million people in the Mexican highlands. The fifteenth- and sixteenth-century Spanish invaders encountered a disease called 'modorro', which some historians believe was typhus. In New England in 1629, however, it was certainly typhus that killed both colonists and natives before spreading steadily eastwards over the next two hundred years.

Controlling the spread of typhus

Navies also suffered badly. However, the eighteenth-century British surgeon James Lind – best known for prescribing the lime juice that prevented another disease, scurvy – ordered that sailors be stripped, scrubbed, shaved and given clean clothes, which ensured British warships stayed largely clear of the typhus-carrying louse.

A breakthrough came in 1910 when Charles Nicolle at the Pasteur Institute in Tunis explained the body louse's role in spreading typhus. In the First World War, the countries fighting on the Western Front introduced delousing and there was not a single outbreak. In the east, however, it was a different story. Serbia saw 150,000 typhus deaths in the first six months of the war, while Russia suffered horribly in the years after the Revolution. In all, there were thirty million cases in the Soviet Union and Eastern Europe between 1918 and 1922, with an estimated three million deaths. Vladimir Lenin, the leader of Soviet Russia, is quoted as saying: 'Either Socialism will defeat the louse, or the louse will defeat Socialism.'

In 1939, the British government began screening Irishmen signing up to fight in the Second World War. Those with lice had their body hair shaved and were made to stand naked in baths while attendants wearing rubber aprons and wellington boots hosed them down with disinfectant. The chief medical officer said their 'shame, fear and outrage' were palpable. However, the principle was sound, even if the method was crude.

In 1943, Italian troops returning from North Africa brought typhus to Naples, where it spread first to the prisoners of war and then to the civilian population. The following year the Nazis discovered

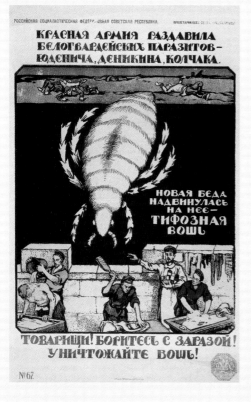

Российская Социалистическая Федеративная Советская Республика.   ПРОЛЕТАРИИ ВСЕХ СТРАН СОЕДИНЯЙТЕСЬ!

КРАСНАЯ АРМИЯ РАЗДАВИЛА БЕЛОГВАРДЕЙСКИХ ПАРАЗИТОВ — ЮДЕНИЧА, ДЕНИКИНА, КОЛЧАКА.

НОВАЯ БЕДА НАДВИНУЛАСЬ НА НЕЕ — ТИФОЗНАЯ ВОШЬ

ТОВАРИЩИ! БОРИТЕСЬ С ЗАРАЗОЙ! УНИЧТОЖАЙТЕ ВОШЬ!

№ 67.

Above: Russian Soviet Federative Socialist Republic poster, 1921. After the defeat of the White Army, a new white peril threatens in the form of the typhus louse.

fourteen-year-old Anne Frank and her family in hiding in Amsterdam. Anne and her sister Margot were sent to Bergen-Belsen concentration camp where they both died of typhus four months later.

The potent insecticide dichloro-diphenyltrichloroethane (DDT) came into use for delousing during the Second World War and was hailed as a wonder preparation. People were sometimes sprayed with it. DDT certainly protected against typhus, but unfortunately it also turned out to be toxic to a far wider range of species than the body louse, including human beings. It is now largely banned across the world, except for a very limited use for malaria control in parts of Africa, where the benefits are thought to outweigh the risks.

Recent outbreaks

In 2006, an employee at a wilderness camp in the US state of Pennsylvania was diagnosed with what is known as sylvatic epidemic typhus, caused by the same organism as louse-borne typhus but linked to close contact with flying squirrels. Three more workers were found to have had the disease in the previous two years. They had slept in the same cabin and had seen or heard flying squirrels inside the wall next to their beds. Until then, only forty-one cases had been recorded in the United States between 1976, when the disease was first recognised, to 2002. Tests on the flying squirrels showed that 71 per cent were infected with *R. prowazekii*. Infected fleas and lice living on the squirrels may be responsible for transmitting the infection to humans but exactly how this happens is not yet understood.

Today epidemic typhus is rare across the globe but persists in the highlands and cold areas of Central and Eastern Africa, Central and South America and Asia. Most of the recent outbreaks have been in Burundi, Ethiopia and Rwanda. In Burundi in 1995, after some years of absence, the disease broke out in Ngozi prison, and then again in 1997, where 760,000 people, displaced by civil war, were living in refugee camps in appalling conditions.

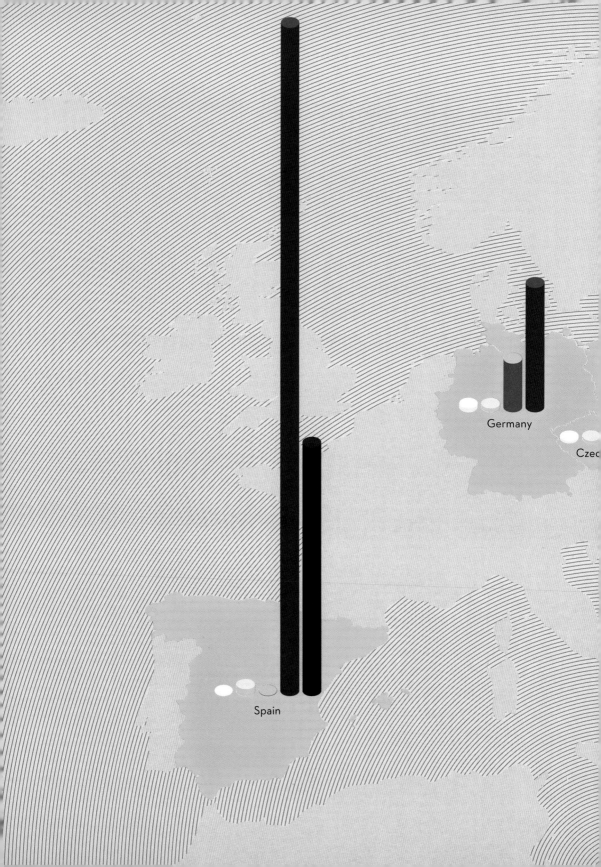

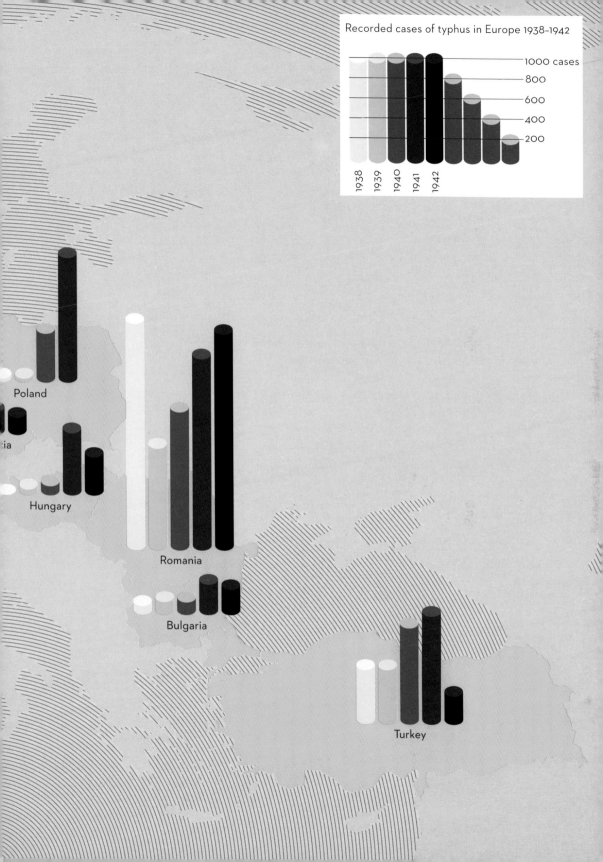

Recorded cases of typhus in Europe 1938–1942

1000 cases
800
600
400
200

1938 1939 1940 1941 1942

Poland

ia

Hungary

Romania

Bulgaria

Turkey

Yellow fever

Causal agent	Virus belonging to the genus Flavivirus
Transmission	Infected mosquitoes
Symptoms	Fever, headache, jaundice, muscle pain, nausea, vomiting and fatigue
Prevalence	Found in tropical and sub-tropical parts of Africa and South America
Incidence and deaths	Not known. One estimate is 84,000–170,000 severe cases and 29,000–60,000 deaths in 2013 but number of cases thought to be hugely under-reported.
Prevention	Vaccination
Treatment	No specific treatment but symptoms treated with drugs
Global strategy	The World Health Organization (WHO) aims to eliminate yellow fever by 2026 through measures including affordable vaccines for at-risk populations and containing outbreaks fast

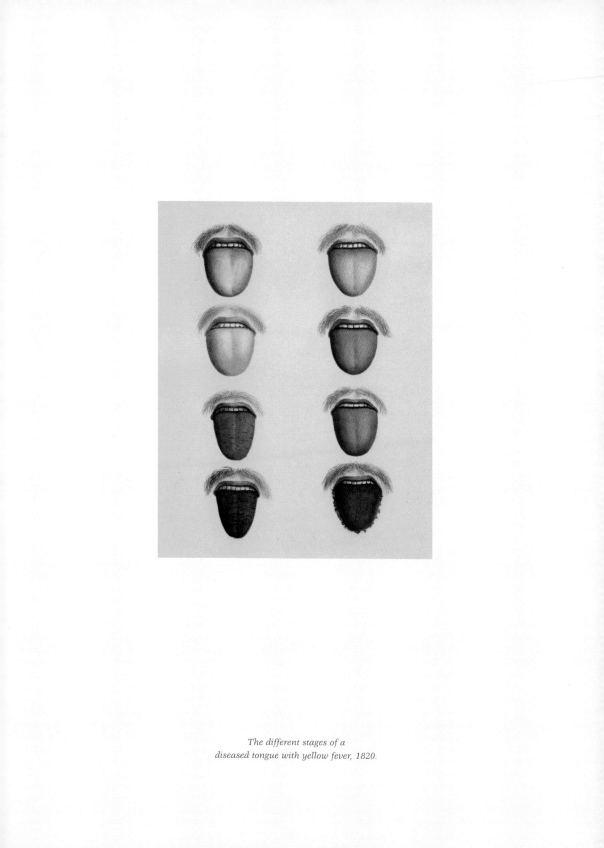

*The different stages of a
diseased tongue with yellow fever, 1820.*

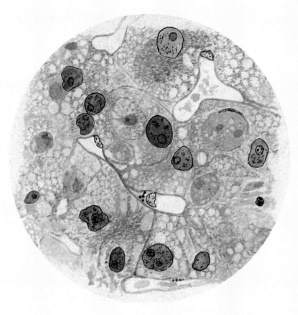

Above: Watercolour depicting a section of the liver
of a patient infected with yellow fever, c. 1920.

In the War Memorial Chapel in Washington National Cathedral, a stained-glass window shows not a saint but a young man with a hypodermic needle and a mosquito. Few people today have heard of Dr Jesse W. Lazear, but he was given this rare commemoration for his sacrifice to medical science.

Lazear was a thirty-four-year-old US army surgeon based in Havana in 1900 and a member of a new commission set up to look into the causes of yellow fever. In the 1898 Spanish-American War, yellow fever killed thousands of US soldiers in Cubout of the nearly three thousand lives lost, less than three hundred men died from their wounds. Finding a way to control the disease shot to the top of the US military agenda.

In 1881, a Cuban doctor, Carlos Finlay, had suggested that yellow fever was spread by mosquitoes. Then his ideas were received with some scepticism but by 1899 scientists had discovered that malaria was spread by mosquitoes, and Finlay was taken more seriously.

The army bacteriologist heading the US commission, Walter Reed, had already disproved one theory: that the infection came from drinking river water. He noticed though that the soldiers who fell sick were in the habit of following a track through some mosquito-infested marshy woodlands at night, while those who avoided the area stayed healthy. So Lazear and his colleague James Carroll decided to put Finlay's ideas to the test, reportedly while their boss, Reed, was away in Washington. They allowed themselves to be bitten by infected mosquitoes. Lazear wrote to his wife: 'I rather think I am on the track of the real germ.' Seventeen days later he was dead. Carroll was very ill but survived.

Reed then set up Camp Lazear, which consisted of some cabins in a remote spot, where he carried out controlled experiments using more human volunteers. He took great care to ensure that his subjects understood what they were agreeing to – which was by no means routine at the time – and produced what is one of the earliest 'informed consent' forms. His results showed that yellow fever was transmitted from a sick person to a healthy one by a bite from an infected mosquito and also that mosquitoes were the only carriers. (Some scientists had suggested that the disease could also be passed on from person to person through direct contact with body fluids.)

Based on these findings, the United States introduced a strict control pro-gramme, spraying mosquitoes, putting screens on buildings and draining swamps. As a result, yellow fever was virtually eliminated, first in Havana and then in Panama, where construction workers on the Panama Canal had suffered badly from both yellow fever and malaria.

From African rainforests to the New World

Little is known of the origins of the disease but the virus responsible is thought to have emerged from the central African rainforests. Over generations, the thinking goes, Africans developed some resistance, which led to it taking the form of a mild childhood illness. However, when European slave traders arrived on the continent in the sixteenth and seventeenth centuries,

Below: A parodic cosmological diagram showing opposing aspects of the life of colonialists in Jamaica; at the bottom we see the hells of yellow fever, c. 1800.

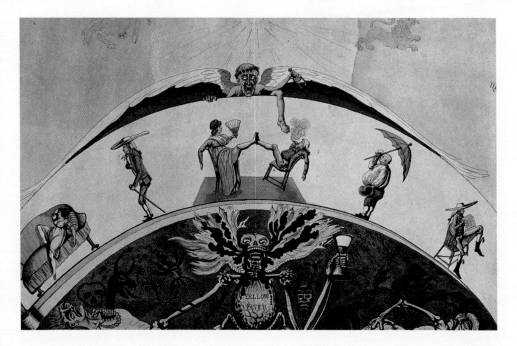

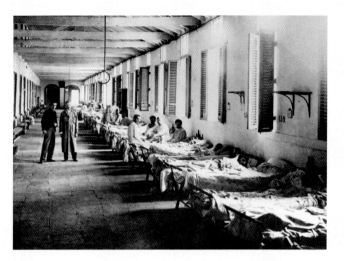

they had no such immunity and for them it proved devastating.

Spanish conquistadors and the slaves then took yellow fever to the Americas. The first recorded epidemic was in Barbados in 1647, and the following year yellow fever broke out in Cuba and on the Yucatan peninsula in southeast Mexico. In 1741, during the strangely named War of Jenkins' Ear, the British admiral besieging Cartagena on the Columbian coast lost a swathe of his fighting force to disease, mainly yellow fever. Estimates vary but range from around eight thousand dead out of twelve thousand men to as much as twenty thousand out of twenty-seven thousand.

By the end of the eighteenth century, the disease was endemic along the east coast of the Americas from Boston down to Rio de Janeiro. An estimated 10 per cent of the residents of Philadelphia died in 1793 and more than one-third of the population fled. New Orleans was hit several times, with an epidemic in 1853 killing an estimated nine thousand, and Memphis was almost abandoned as being uninhabitable after devastating outbreaks in 1878 and 1879. By then the disease was known as yellow jack, partly because one of the symptoms was a yellow tinge to the skin, due to jaundice, but also because ships displayed a warning yellow flag when they came into port with victims on board.

Ports on Europe's western seaboard – Lisbon, St Nazaire and Swansea – were also attacked. In an outbreak in Swansea in 1865, the mosquitoes are thought to have arrived on a ship from Cuba during a spell of exceptionally hot weather. Over the next twenty-five days, at least twenty-seven people fell sick and fifteen of them died.

Yellow fever usually sparked panic due to its terrible symptoms and high death rate. In 1897, a man in Memphis wrote a dreadful description of the death of a young girl, possibly his niece, which began: 'Lucille died at ten o'clock Tuesday night after such suffering as I hope never to witness ... The poor girl's screams might be heard for half a square.' One feature of the disease is that gastric acid turns the

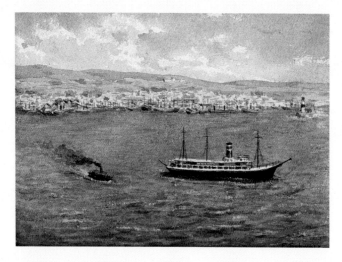

stomach contents black and so the victim's vomit resembles coffee grains, hence the Spanish name *vomito negro*, or 'black vomit'. Yellow fever was also known as stranger's disease because a newcomer often triggered an outbreak.

Before its mode of transmission was understood, the widely held belief was that yellow fever was caused by miasma, the foul smells emanating from filth, combined with hot, humid weather. In the Philadelphia outbreak, a pile of rotting coffee beans was thought to be the culprit. But not everyone was convinced. A doctor in nineteenth-century New Orleans remarked: 'We have heat and moisture, dead dogs, cats and chickens all over the streets and plenty of hungry doctors, yet yellow jack will not come.'

Different habitats, different species

The yellow fever virus is transmitted by two species of mosquito that live in different habitats: some breed around dwellings (domestic), others in the jungle (wild), and some in both settings (semi-domestic). Once infected, a mosquito remains so for life. There are three types of transmission cycle. Sylvatic, or jungle, yellow fever occurs in tropical rainforests. Here, the main host, or primary reservoir, are monkeys. After a wild mosquito bites an infected monkey, the insect passes the virus on to other monkeys through its bite. Occasionally, humans working or travelling in the forest are bitten and become sick.

In intermediate yellow fever, semi-domestic mosquitoes, which breed both in the wild and around houses, infect both monkeys and people. Greater contact between people and the infected mosquitoes leads to increased transmission, and many villages can experience outbreaks at the same time. This is the most common type of outbreak in Africa.

The third type of transmission, and the one responsible for the large epidemics, is known as urban yellow fever. This occurs when infected people introduce the virus into heavily populated areas that have a high density of mosquitoes and where most people have little or no immunity. In these conditions, infected mosquitoes transmit the virus from person to person.

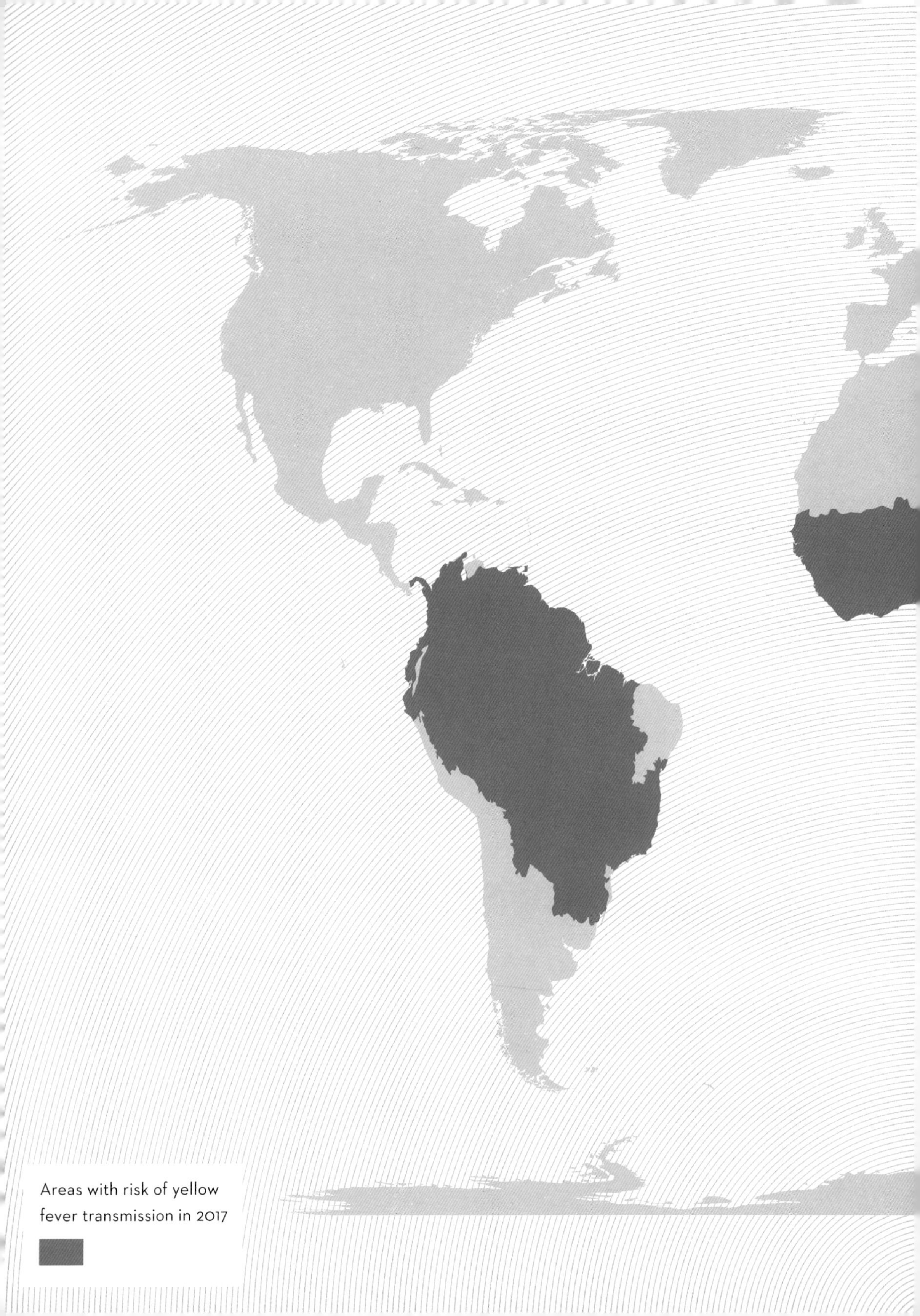
Areas with risk of yellow
fever transmission in 2017

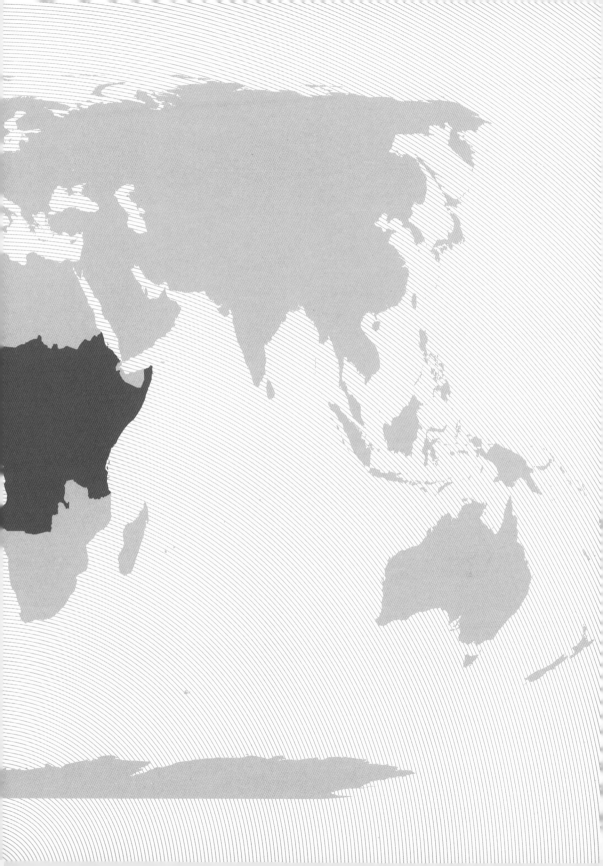

Yellow fever in the twenty-first century

The virus remains endemic in tropical areas of Africa and Central and South America: in 2013, there were an estimated 84,000 to 170,000 severe cases and 29,000 to 60,000 deaths. No one knows how many people around the world contract the disease today, but it is thought to be hugely under-reported, with the true numbers as much as 10 to 250 times the official figures.

However, progress has been made in controlling the disease. In 2006, the World Health Organization (WHO) launched an initiative to ensure that the vaccine, which is safe, effective and cheap, was available everywhere.

The development of that vaccine had proved a long and complex business and pushed the then state of scientific knowledge to its limits. For many years, starting in the 1930s, two vaccines were available: one – produced at the US Rockefeller Foundation – was used in most of the West and the another – developed in Britain and the Pasteur Institute in France – was used in France and its African colonies. But since 1982, just one vaccine, known as 17D, has been in use.

By 2016, more than 105 million people in West Africa had been vaccinated and no outbreaks were reported in the region during 2015. However, over a six-month period to January 2018, 35 cases were reported in Brazil, including 20 deaths, while 145 suspected cases were under investigation.

The *Aedes aegypti* mosquito, which carries urban yellow fever, was at one point eliminated from most of Central and South America through rigorous control programmes. Dichlorodiphenyltrichloro-ethane, the first modern synthetic insecticide and more commonly known as DDT, was introduced in the 1940s. It proved highly effective in controlling the insect. According to the Pan American Health Organization, the *A. aegypti* mosquito was eradicated from twenty-two countries in the Americas. In the 1960s, however, concerns started to be raised about the damage that DDT was doing to the environment as well as the risk it posed to human health. In 2004, the Stockholm Convention on Persistent Organic Pollutants came into force, a global treaty banning DDT except for controlling malaria in parts of Africa.

The *A. aegypti* mosquito has now re-emerged in urban areas. Attempts to tackle it include using insecticides that target the mosquito larvae at the insect's breeding sites such as water storage containers and wherever standing water collects. However, control programmes are not a practical way of tackling wild mosquitoes in the forests.

The WHO says that prompt detection followed by mass emergency vaccination is essential. The organisation recommends that every country at risk has at least one laboratory capable of carrying out basic diagnostic tests: just one laboratory-confirmed case in an unvaccinated population is classed as an outbreak. Occasionally, a traveller brings yellow fever into a disease-free country, so many countries now ask for proof of vaccination before granting entry.

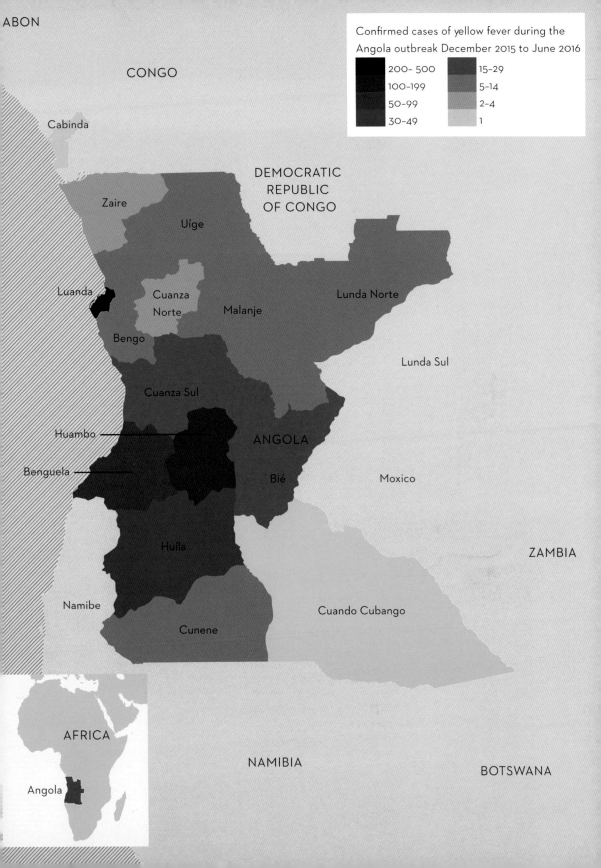

Zika

||||||||||||||

Causal agent	Zika virus
Transmission	Mainly bite from infected mosquito but also person to person through sexual contact
Symptoms	Include fever, skin rash, conjunctivitis, muscle and joint pain, malaise, headache. The virus can trigger the neurological disorder Guillain-Barré syndrome and in pregnant women can lead to microcephaly in the child.
Prevalence	Parts of Africa, Asia, the Caribbean, South and Central America, Mexico and the Pacific Islands
Prevention	Avoidance of mosquito bites and of sexual transmission. Use of insecticides during outbreaks.
Treatment	No treatment for the virus but symptoms are treated with drugs
Global strategy	Surveillance in endemic areas to ensure fast detection of cases and containment of outbreaks. Destruction of mosquito breeding sites and reduction of contact with mosquitoes.

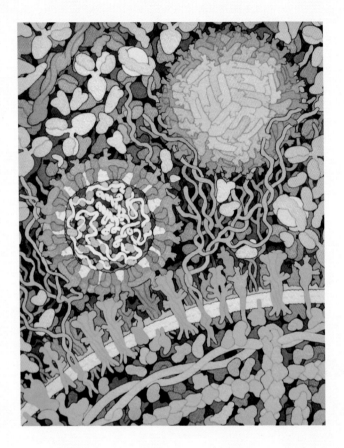

*Illustration depicting a cross-section
of the zika virus.*

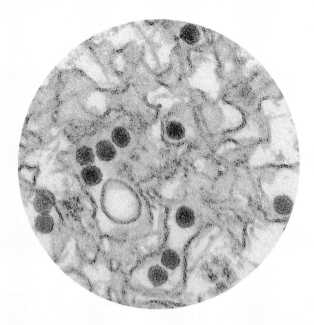

Above: *Microscopic image of zika virus particles.*

Mayara Santos de Oliveira was sixteen when she gave birth to Alejandro, her 'special' baby. If she had a fever, a rash or muscle ache during her pregnancy, she didn't think them important. A campaigner for women's rights in Brazil commented that people like Mayara had lived with tropical diseases such as dengue, chikungunya and malaria for a long time. Women had told her: 'I felt some pain [in pregnancy] but nothing different from everyday life.'

Emergence of a new strain

In 2015, a disease previously considered benign metamorphosed without warning into a global health emergency. Back in 2007, after sixty years of seeming inactivity, zika broke out briefly on Yap Island in Micronesia in the western Pacific. But while an estimated five thousand people were infected – more than 70 per cent of the island's population – no one was hospitalised and no one died. Scientists thought that perhaps a new strain of the virus had emerged with more potential to cause an epidemic. The same had happened in the 1970s when the dengue virus – related to the zika virus and spread by the same species of mosquito – had begun island-hopping around the Pacific.

The next surprise was more worrying. Zika broke out again in 2013–14, this time in French Polynesia, striking seven islands and infecting around thirty thousand people. As before there were no deaths, but the disease had clearly established a strong foothold in the Pacific and public health experts decided that it no longer looked so harmless.

During and after this outbreak, patients began presenting with some usually rare complications, including forty-two cases of a severe neurological disorder called Guillain-Barré syndrome – a twenty-fold increase over previous years – sixteen of which had to be admitted to intensive care. However, the dengue virus, which had previously been linked to Guillain-Barré, was also present in the region, so the scientists couldn't be sure if zika was involved.

Zika reaches Brazil

The big shift though came when zika struck in Brazil. The infection was almost certainly brought into the country by a traveller from French Polynesia, as the viruses from the two countries were virtually identical. At first, epidemiologists thought that the cause lay with the influx of visitors for the 2014 World Cup football competition, held in Brazil in June and July, but no teams from countries with a zika outbreak had taken part. Then attention switched to the World Sprint Championship canoe race held in Rio de Janeiro in August, which included competitors from four Pacific Island countries with active zika, including French Polynesia.

In fact, while the first confirmed case is dated to May 2015, later studies placed the virus's entry to 2013. Further work indicated cases in Haiti as early as December 2014, although the outbreak was not detected until 2016. The French Polynesia virus appears to have entered the Americas by way of Easter island.

Spreading throughout Latin America

Once it had established a foothold in Brazil, zika spread fast throughout the country and then Latin America and the Caribbean. Within a year, the virus was in nearly every country or territory infested with *Aedes aegypti*, the main species of mosquito that transmits zika as well as yellow fever and dengue. Two factors helped trigger the explosion: the lack of immunity among populations and the habits of the mosquito.

The *A. aegypti* mosquito is known as the 'gothic cockroach of mosquitoes' because of its liking for the colour black. The World Health Organization (WHO) describes it as the ultimate 'citified' mosquito because it has adapted to life in those tropical areas that have seen rapid and sprawling urbanisation. It flourishes in litter, open ditches, clogged drains, water storage containers, tyre dumps and crowded buildings: wherever the infrastructure – provision of clean running water and sewers, for example – has failed to keep pace with the growth of the population. The insect can breed in a discarded bottle cap or plastic wrapper.

In July 2015, Brazil reported an increase in neurological disorders including Guillain-Barré mainly in the northeast of the country, which was the early epicentre for the zika outbreak. This pattern would later be repeated in other countries that experienced large outbreaks, including Colombia, the Dominican Republic, El Salvador and Venezuela.

Zika linked to microcephaly

In October, another report from Brazil highlighted a new concern: fifty-four cases of microcephaly were diagnosed among newborn babies since August. In microcephaly, the baby's head is abnormally small and the brain underdeveloped, meaning the child is likely to have severe learning difficulties. The news of a possible link between this

First recorded incidence of zika virus
around the globe

1947		January 2015
1948		February 2015
1954		April 2015
1960–1983		July 2015
2007–2009		October 2015
2012–2014		November 2015
		December 2015
		January 2016
		February 2016

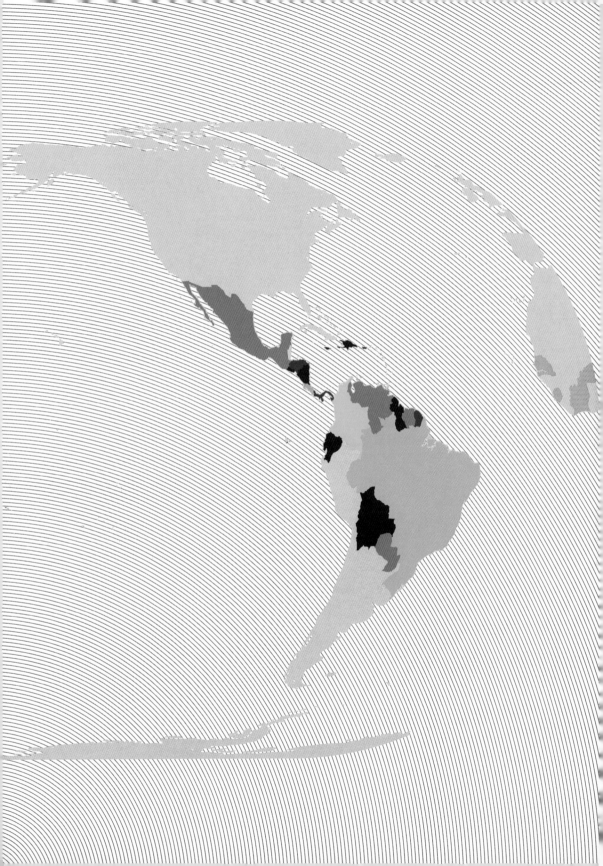

condition and zika virus in pregnant women astounded scientists and sparked a worldwide panic. The experts looked again at French Polynesia and found at least seventeen babies with various severe brain malformations including microcephaly born during or in the aftermath of that outbreak.

When more research in January 2016 showed a convincing a link between zika and Guillain-Barré, the WHO immediately designated the situation a Public Health Emergency of International Concern. In April, the US Centers for Disease Control and Prevention established beyond doubt a link between zika infection in pregnancy and microcephaly in newborn infants.

The WHO says that the emergence of zika in the Americas 'surprised a world that was ill-prepared to cope, especially with the heart-breaking neurological abnormalities in newborns'. And with no vaccine, there was nothing to offer women of child-bearing age except advice about avoiding mosquito bites, delaying pregnancy and not travelling to areas with active transmission of the virus.

And then there is the cost of care. In Brazil, many women giving birth to babies with what is known as congenital zika syndrome – microcephaly and a ranging of other disabling conditions – are young and poor. In a rich country, the costs of caring for a single child with microcephaly have been estimated at as high as ten million US dollars. In a poor country, the WHO warns, the burden of care will largely fall on mothers who may have to give up work and may find it hard to get support from health and social services.

Complacency leads to outbreaks
Unlike yellow fever and malaria, it is not only mosquitoes that spread zika. Before the Brazil outbreak it was already known that the virus could also be passed on through sexual contact, but this mode of transmission turned out to be more common than previously thought.

Zika, the WHO says, has particular implications for the countries in the outbreak zone, all of which have large percentages of their populations in poverty. In terms of transmission, few of these countries offer universal access to sexual health and family planning services, and a recent study showed that countries in Latin America and the Caribbean had the highest proportion (56 per cent) of unintended pregnancies anywhere in the world. The high number of unplanned pregnancies is partly linked to religious belief, and in February 2016 Pope Francis caused controversy when he suggested that contraceptives could be used to help prevent the spread of zika. Avoiding pregnancy was not an 'absolute evil', he said.

In tropical cities throughout the developing world, many people cannot afford air-conditioning, window screens or even insect repellents. With no piped water and poor sanitation, they are forced to store water in containers, providing ideal conditions for the mosquitoes.

The WHO puts some of the blame for the rise in zika on what it claims is the complacency that set in after the huge success of mosquito control efforts in the 1940s and 1950s. With yellow fever apparently conquered, the funding for mosquito control dried up, the organisation claims. Its response shifted from prevention as the first line of defence to surveillance to pick up early signs of an outbreak and then mounting an emergency response.

The weaknesses of this stopgap approach have been shown by the dramatic resurgence of dengue, the recent emergence of chikungunya – a fever with generalised symptoms – as a significant threat to health, the delayed detection and subsequent exponential spread of ebola in West Africa, and the return of urban yellow fever to Africa. Zika, says WHO, 'seems destined to make these weaknesses even more explicit'.

Still a lot to learn

Despite a mass of research following the Brazil epidemic – and in 2018 there was another outbreak there – zika is still poorly understood. It is known to have been in parts of Asia and Africa for several decades, but what level of immunity, if any, has this conferred on different populations?

In Africa, the transmission pattern is what is known as a sylvatic cycle, involving forest mosquitoes that feed on monkeys. This may mean that historically there have been very few human cases. It is also possible though that cases have been missed because the vast majority of zika infections are symptom free and any symptoms that do occur are mild and similar to those of dozens of other common tropical viral infections.

Urgent research is underway, focusing on some complex questions about, for example, the different lineages of the

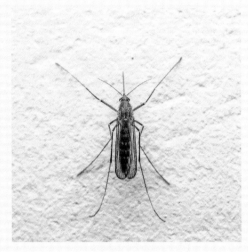

Above: *The zika virus is commonly transmitted from the bite of an infected mosquito.*

virus, the levels of immunity in populations and the virus's likely future paths of travel. In terms of prevention, scientists are looking at a bacterium called *Wolbachia pipientis*, found naturally in insects throughout the world. Wolbachia are known to protect fruit flies from viruses, so perhaps they could protect the *A. azegypti* mosquito from those viruses that cause disease in human beings.

The situation is now dramatically different from when, quite recently, zika was seen as essentially harmless and not worth much time or trouble.

French Polynesia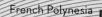

Spread of zika virus during
the 2013–16 outbreak

	Point of origin
	2013
	2014
	2015

| January 2016 |
| February 2016 |
| March 2016 |
| April 2016 |
| May 2016 |
| June 2016 |
| July 2016 |
| August 2016 |

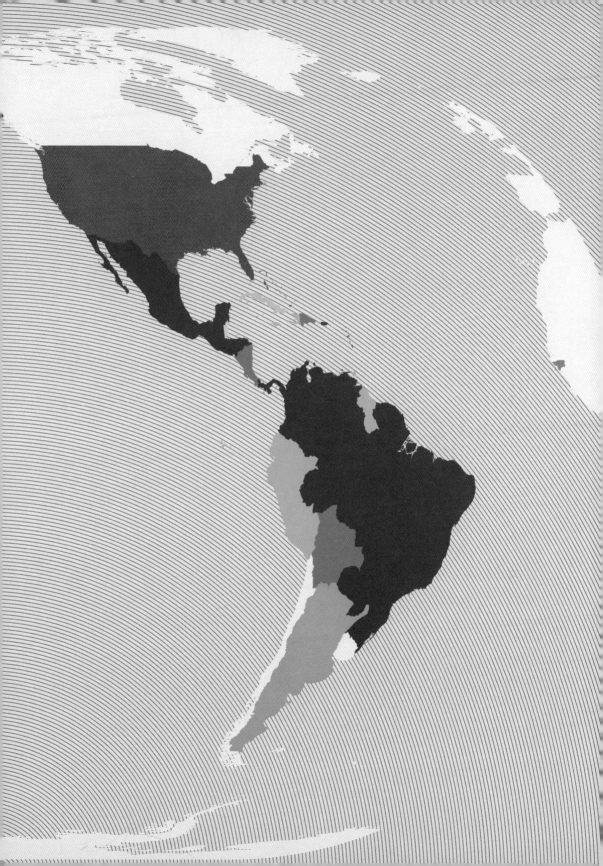

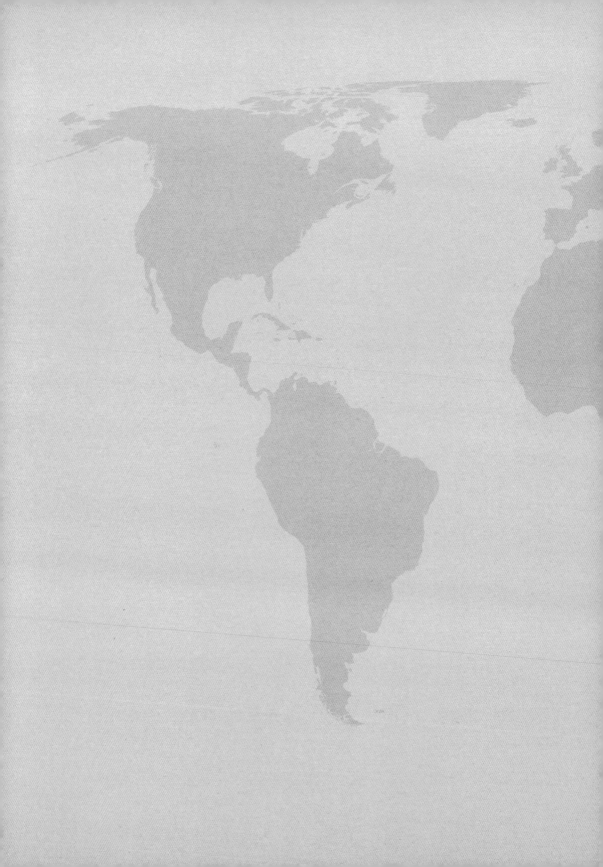

SECTION 4
HUMAN
TO HUMAN

Polio

|||||||||||||||||||

Causal agent	Three strains of wild polio virus but type 2 now eliminated
Transmission	Person to person via the oral-faecal route
Symptoms	Usually symptomless but symptoms include stiffness in the neck and back, abnormal reflexes and difficulty swallowing and breathing. In rare cases leads to paralysis
Incidence and deaths	22 reported cases in 2017
Prevalence	Only endemic now in Nigeria, Pakistan and Afghanistan
Prevention	Vaccination
Treatment	No treatment for the virus but symptoms relieved with a range of drugs and therapies.
Global strategy	Mass vaccination of children. In 2017, the World Health Organization (WHO) believed the complete eradication of polio was well within our grasp

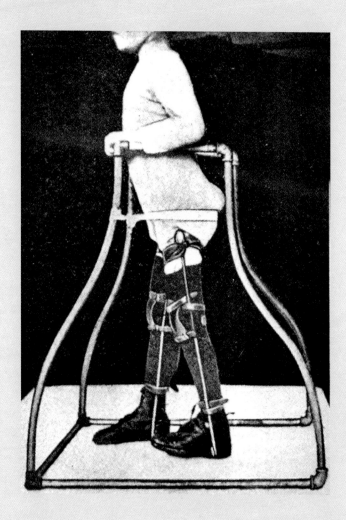

The treatment of polio with the use of
a walking frame from R.W. Lovett's
Treatment of Infantile Paralysis, *1917.*

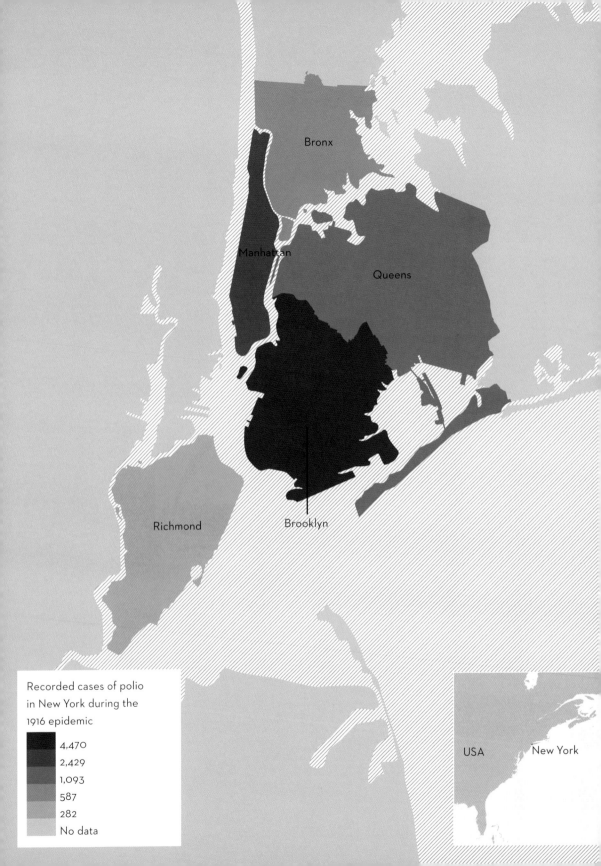

Bronx

Manhattan

Queens

Richmond

Brooklyn

Recorded cases of polio
in New York during the
1916 epidemic

4,470
2,429
1,093
587
282
No data

USA   New York

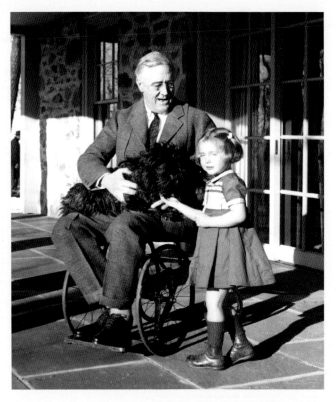

On the 17 June 1916, the authorities in New York's Brooklyn County announced another outbreak of a disease that appeared from time to time, usually affecting a small number of people in a small locality. This time though it would turn out rather differently.

Fleeing New York's epidemic

Poliomyelitis spread fast and wide, first through the city, then out into the surrounding areas and finally across the country. In New York, there was widespread panic. Thousands fled the city. Cinemas were closed, public gatherings cancelled and amusement parks, swimming pools and beaches lay deserted. The names and addresses of the victims were published every day in the press, placards were displayed on their houses and their families quarantined.

Inspectors were posted at railway stations and at boat landings along the Delaware River, turning away all children under sixteen trying to cross into the state of Pennsylvania without a certificate of health. *The New York Times* described a more personal and distressing incident:

> Unable to obtain a physician, he [the father] put the boy into an automobile and drove to the Smith Infirmary, but the child died on the way and the doctors at the hospital would not receive the body ... He drove around Staten Island with the boy's body for hours looking for someone who would receive it.

By the time the epidemic was over, there had been more than nine thousand cases and 2,343 deaths in New York and twenty-seven thousand cases and six thousand deaths nationwide. Most of the victims were children under five. Over the next forty years, the disease broke out with increasing frequency and increasing deadliness. At its peak in the 1940s and 1950s, polio was paralysing or killing over half a million people worldwide every year.

Previous local outbreaks

Until the 1880s, polio had been a rare condition, but by the mid-twentieth century it was causing epidemics across the globe. Early brief reports describe what appear to be small and very local outbreaks, including one on St Helena, an island in the South Atlantic, and one in Worksop in England in the 1830s. From the 1880s reports of other small local outbreaks, usually with fewer than thirty cases, began to emerge more frequently in Europe. Then in the early 1900s, larger epidemics hit Norway with nine hundred cases and Sweden with one thousand.

Polio, which causes inflammation of the meninges – the membrane covering the brain and spinal chord – appears to have been attacking human beings for millennia. An Egyptian stone slab from about 1400 BC is engraved with the image of a young priest with a shortened foot, taking the weight of the left side of his body by balancing on his toes. His deformity is typical of poliomyelitis. Other illustrations show children walking with sticks and otherwise healthy-looking people with withered limbs.

Claudius, the first-century AD Roman Emperor, who famously walked with a limp, is thought to have been a likely victim, as is the eighteenth-century writer Sir Walter Scott. As a child in 1773, Scott developed 'a severe teething fever which deprived him of the power of his right leg', which modern medical practitioners believe could have been polio.

In Scott's time, doctors knew nothing of polio as a specific condition and called it by a variety of names, including dental paralysis, infantile spinal paralysis, essential paralysis of children, myelitis of the anterior horns, tephromyelitis and paralysis of the morning. The first and most influential medical description that established polio as a separate disease came in 1840 from the German orthopaedic surgeon Jakob Heine, and the Swedish physician Karl Oskar Medin described its epidemic nature in 1890. For some time after, polio was also known as as Heine-Medin disease.

Sudden increase in cases

But after surviving quietly in the environment for thousands of years, why, in the first half of the twentieth century, did the poliovirus break its boundaries and emerge as a mass killer? There are countless theories, based on a range of social, environmental, biological and demographic factors. They include an increased virulence in the virus and/or in its ability to cause infection, as well as changes in human nutrition. However, hygiene and its link with immunity has been a key focus for researchers.

Ironically, at a time when decent sanitation in Europe and the United States was defeating some of the great killer diseases of the nineteenth century, the blame for the explosion in polio has been levelled at decent drains and clean drinking water.

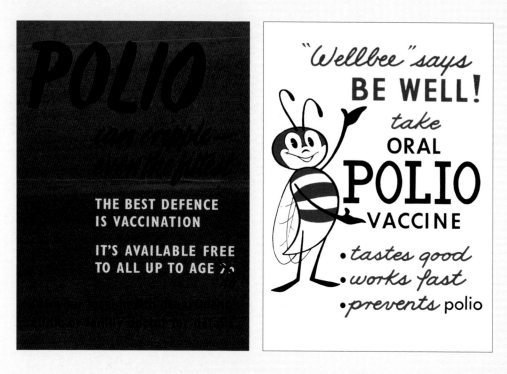

Above: *British Ministry of Health poster for the vaccination against polio, c. 1940.*

Above: *Centers for Disease Control poster, in which their symbol of public health, 'Wellbee', encourages people to take the polio vaccine, 1963.*

Poliovirus, which is highly contagious, is mainly spread through infected faeces. One theory is that by removing that faecal contamination from drinking water, babies in early infancy had less exposure to poliovirus, so reducing immunity among the population.

Polio differs from many other epidemic diseases in that around 95 per cent of those infected have no symptoms at all. Another major difference is that those who recover can be left with permanent and severe disabilities, although less than 2 per cent of people who contract polio become paralysed. If paralysis affects the throat and chest, however, the patient is at risk of suffocating.

Improvements for polio patients

In 1928, Phillip Drinker at Harvard University in Massachusetts, invented a device for treating respiratory paralysis consisting of an airtight wooden box with a motor-driven bellows. In 2017, seventy-year-old Paul Alexander in Texas, who caught polio in 1952 when he was six, described how he had spent most of his life in his 'iron lung', answering the phone and typing by means of a plastic wand attached to his mouth. Despite his handicap, Mr Alexander qualified as a lawyer, taking his iron lung with him to law school. In 2017, it was not known how many other polio survivors with respiratory paralysis were still alive, trapped in their machines, but

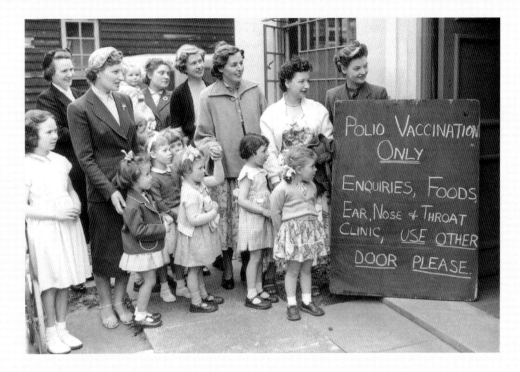

their number was thought to be down to just a handful.

The 1916 New York epidemic was not only the impetus for developments in artificial ventilation but for huge advancements in medical science and rehabilitation therapy, as well as changes in social attitudes. The hunt for a vaccine began immediately, with massive fund-raising to support the research. The first vaccine, administered by injection, became available in 1955 and an oral version followed in 1959, developed through a US–Soviet collaboration. Mass trials of the oral vaccine in the Soviet Union and Eastern Europe in 1959–60 ensured that most of that region was quickly polio-free.

At the same time, many people who had been disabled by polio came out of hospital to face both physical barriers in their everyday life and also discrimination.

Above: A group of mothers with their children waiting outside a clinic in Middlesex, UK, for the first polio vaccinations to begin, 1956.

Their battle for access and equality resulted in the legacy of modern rehabilitation therapy and the disability rights movement, with disability seen not simply in medical terms but as a social and civil rights issue.

Franklin D. Roosevelt, the US President from 1933 to 1945, was diagnosed with polio in 1921 when he was thirty-nine and left unable to walk, although some experts now question that diagnosis. Roosevelt founded the National Foundation for Infantile Paralysis to combat polio. Now known as the March of Dimes, the organisation works today to combat birth defects, premature birth and infant mortality. Designers meanwhile turned

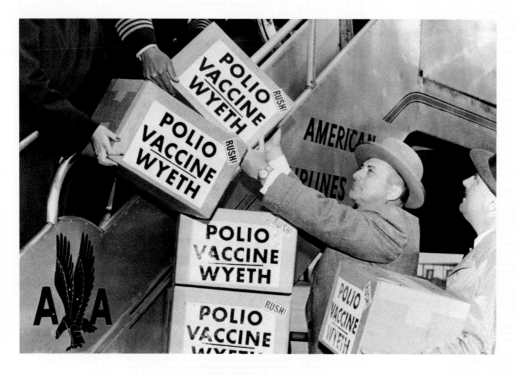

Above: Boxes of the polio vaccine being shipped to Europe, 1955.

their attention to helping disabled people live a more active and rewarding life, with specially designed aids and vehicles and better access to public buildings such as colleges and theatres and to transport systems.

An end to a killer?

Widespread vaccination programmes saw the number of polio cases fall globally between 1974 and 1994 from around fifty million to under five million. In 1988, the World Health Assembly launched the Global Polio Eradication Initiative, aimed at eradicating the disease by immunising every child. In 1994, the WHO declared its Americas regions polio-free, followed by the Western Pacific in 2000, Europe in 2002 and Southeast Asia in 2014. This meant that 80 per cent of the world's population were now living in certified polio-free areas. As a result, more than sixteen million people are able to walk today who would otherwise have been paralysed, the WHO claims.

As part of the campaign in war-torn areas, the organisers introduced what they called 'days of tranquillity', when combatants were persuaded to allow teams in to vaccinate children. By the end of 2017 polio was endemic only in Afghanistan, Nigeria and Pakistan, with an occasional spread into neighbouring countries, and WHO believes that the world eradication of this disease is now firmly in sight.

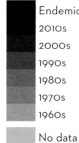

Last recorded case of paralytic
polio around the globe

Endemic today
2010s
2000s
1990s
1980s
1970s
1960s

No data

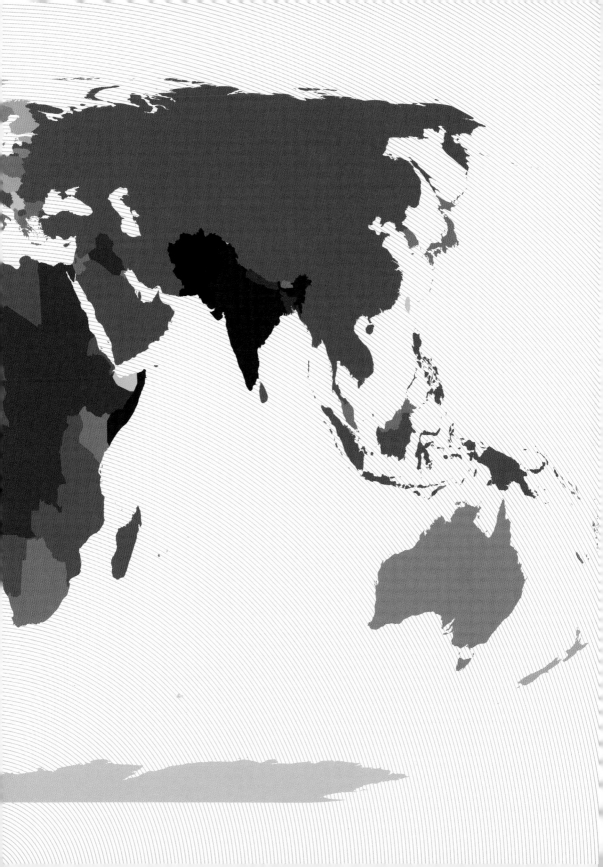

Ebola

||||||||||||||||||||

Causal agent	The ebola virus. Five species identified so far.
Transmission	Transmitted to humans by wild animals, then spreads from person to person through body fluids
Symptoms	Fever, severe headache, muscle pain, weakness, fatigue, diarrhoea, vomiting, abdominal pain, haemorrhaging
Incidence and deaths	28,616 cases in the 2014–16 epidemic and 11,310 deaths. Average case fatality rate is around 50 per cent.
Prevalence	Two isolated outbreaks in the Democratic Republic of the Congo since the global pandemic of 2014–16
Prevention	In affected areas, avoid contact with: body fluids; infected medical equipment and bedding, and bats and non-human primates and bush meat from these animals
Treatment	No proven treatment but treatments for different symptoms and support to maintain the body's functions
Global strategy	Fast containment of outbreaks combined with health education for health workers and general population

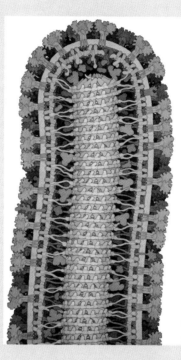

*An illustration of a cross-section
through an ebola virus particle.*

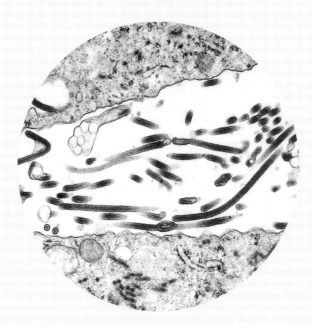

Above: *Microscopic image of the ebola virus.*

The first officially recorded case of the viral disease ebola is that of a Flemish nun called Sister Beata. She died in a clinic in Kinshasa in what is now the Democratic Republic of Congo (DRC) in September 1976, after suffering horrible symptoms including massive haemorrhaging. A few days later, the nun who had taken Sister Beata to hospital fell ill with the same symptoms. She, too, was admitted to the clinic and she too died. She was followed by a young nurse who had been caring for her.

An unknown virus

As Sister Beata lay dying, samples of her blood were sent to a research laboratory in Antwerp for testing because her condition made no sense. The doctors had diagnosed 'yellow fever with haemorrhagic manifestations' but her yellow fever vaccinations were up to date and haemorrhaging is rare in yellow fever.

It turned out that the three women in Kinshasa were not the only cases. Several other nuns at the remote Yambuku mission post in Equateur, along the river Congo, where Sister Beata was based, had already died, seemingly from the same disease. They too had been vaccinated against yellow fever.

The Antwerp scientists began work on the blood samples, looking for antibodies – produced by the body in fighting infection – against yellow fever and several other epidemic diseases, including Lassa fever, a viral infection fairly common in parts of West Africa, and typhoid, a bacterial infection most usually found in Asia, Africa, Latin America and Eastern Europe. The tests all proved negative.

But when the team looked at tissue samples under an electron microscope, they saw worm-like structures, huge compared to most viruses, and previously unknown. They were nothing at all like yellow fever, but they bore some resemblance to another deadly haemorrhagic disease called Marburg, which is indigenous to Africa. Marburg had been identified only nine years earlier in Germany when pharmaceutical workers became ill after handling monkeys imported from Uganda. Seven of the twenty-five people directly infected by the monkeys died and six more fell sick after contact with the victims. By then the mysterious Yambuku outbreak had been raging for three weeks, killing at least two hundred people.

The World Health Organization (WHO) ordered the Antwerp scientists to send their samples to the British government's research laboratory at Porton Down and six days later to the world's reference laboratory for haemorrhagic viruses at the US Centers for Disease Control and Prevention (CDC) in Atlanta, Georgia. Three weeks after Sister Beata's death, the CDC announced the discovery of a new and deadly virus, later named ebola after a river near the mission in Yambuku.

Since then, five strains of the ebola virus have been identified. Four of them cause disease in humans: ebola virus (*Zaire ebolavirus*), the Yambuku strain and the most deadly; Sudan virus (*Sudan ebolavirus*); Taï Forest virus (*Taï Forest ebolavirus*); and Bundibugyo virus (*Bundibugyo ebolavirus*). The fifth, Reston virus (*Reston ebolavirus*), has caused disease in non-human primates such as monkeys and pigs, but not people.

Detecting how ebola spreads

After the first case was detected, Western countries immediately scrambled to put together teams of epidemiologists and virologists to find out all they could about this frightening new disease. Their priority was to discover how it was spreading, which involved what is known as a 'shoe leather' investigation. In other words, the scientists

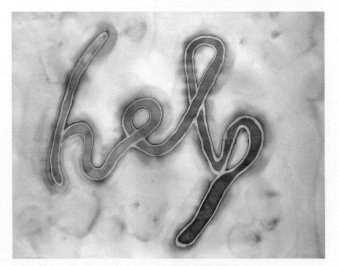

Left: Artistic interpretation of an ebola virus particle, shaped to spell the word 'help'.

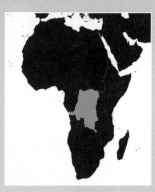

Sudan

Democratic
Republic of the
Congo

Reported cases of ebola
in South Sudan, 1976

████ 284 cases
████ 280 cases

would examine how the disease behaved on the ground and try to identify some common factors among the victims that might throw light on its mode of transmission. By the time they reached Yambuku, fifty-four more people had died. The total was eventually 280, a death rate of 88 per cent.

The mission at the heart of the outbreak was orderly and immaculate, with a courtyard and fringed by palm trees and lawns, next to a small church. As the team approached it, someone shouted: 'Don't come any nearer or you will die like us'. The surviving nuns had holed themselves up in a little guesthouse awaiting death. They had read about a *cordon sanitaire* and had interpreted it literally: a rope was strung around the house and a sign instructed visitors to ring a bell and leave messages at the foot of a tree. By then nine out of seventeen hospital staff had died, as well as thirty-nine people from the sixty families living at the mission, four nuns and two priests.

After the experts questioned local people – collecting data about who had died, when and under what circumstances – they decided that ebola was unlikely to be airborne. Some more intimate form of contact appeared to be required. This was welcome news because airborne diseases such as measles and influenza are, of course, the most contagious.

Over the next few days, two significant factors emerged. First, the investigators noticed what appeared to be a link with funerals. Again and again, the funeral of an ebola victim was followed about a week later by a batch of new cases among the mourners. According to local custom, a corpse is cleaned by family members working barehanded and involves washing all of the body's orifices. The ceremony itself then lasts for several days, during which large numbers of people come together in close contact.

Another clue was that almost all of the early victims among the villagers were pregnant women who had been given vitamin injections at the mission hospital's antenatal clinic. The nuns boiled the glass hypodermics every morning but not for long enough to sterilise them properly. They then reused them all day, with just a quick rinse in sterile water between patients.

All of this suggested that ebola was being passed on through bodily fluids: blood, urine, faeces, saliva, semen and vaginal fluids. It turned out that ebola was relatively difficult to catch. Only those involved in caring for an infected person or in a close relationship – particularly a sexual one – with them, were at risk. Once it was understood how ebola was spreading, prevention was possible. However, health workers on the ground met with considerable hostility when trying to enforce precautions that went against local traditions, most notably in the way funerals were conducted.

In 2014, however, the emphasis on funerals was questioned on the basis that, on the then-available data, the rituals could not be separated from caring for people in late-stage ebola as a possible source of disease transmission.

The scientist who identified the ebola virus, Professor Peter Piot, said that the infection caused epidemics only if basic hospital hygiene was not respected. It was really a disease of poverty and neglect of health systems, he believed. The 'heroic and well-meaning sisters in Yambuku' had shown dramatically that doing good was

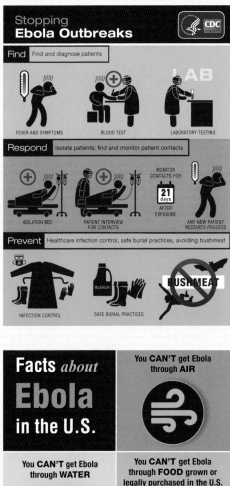

Stopping
Ebola Outbreaks

Find — Find and diagnose patients

FEVER AND SYMPTOMS | BLOOD TEST | LABORATORY TESTING | LAB

Respond — Isolate patients; find and monitor patient contacts

ISOLATION BED | PATIENT INTERVIEW FOR CONTACTS | MONITOR CONTACTS FOR 21 days AFTER EXPOSURE | ANY NEW PATIENT RESTARTS PROCESS

Prevent — Healthcare infection control, safe burial practices, avoiding bushmeat

INFECTION CONTROL | SAFE BURIAL PRACTICES | BUSHMEAT

Facts *about*
Ebola
in the U.S.

You **CAN'T** get Ebola through **AIR**

You **CAN'T** get Ebola through **WATER**

You **CAN'T** get Ebola through **FOOD** grown or legally purchased in the U.S.

You can only get Ebola from
- The body fluids of a person who is sick with or has died from Ebola.
- Objects contaminated with body fluids of a person sick with Ebola or who has died from Ebola.
- Infected fruit bats and primates (apes and monkeys).
- And, possibly from contact with semen from a man who has recovered from Ebola (for example, by having oral, vaginal, or anal sex).

not enough, and it could actually be dangerous if it were not bedded in technical competence and sound evidence. 'Health, economic and social development are unmistakably intertwined', he added.

Global panic

Sister Beata in the DRC is the first officially recorded case, but three months before she died a haemorrhagic fever broke out among factory workers in Nzara (in what is now South Sudan), which borders the DRC to the north. There were 284 cases between June and November 1976 and 151 people died. The disease was later identified as ebola and, although the link is not clear, Nzara is thought to be a possible source for the DRC outbreak.

Since 1976, the disease has broken out regularly in Africa, particularly in the DRC and Uganda. Because it often occurs in isolated, poorly populated areas, it is believed that it sometimes goes unrecorded.

From 1989 to 1994, there were four isolated incidences of the Reston virus strain in laboratories in developed countries, including the United States and Italy. However, these incidents were all linked to laboratories where monkeys used for research were found to be carrying the virus. In two incidents, no humans, only monkeys, were involved, and in the others, laboratory workers had antibodies to the virus but no symptoms of the disease.

Then in March 2014, everything changed. Ebola struck in West Africa, where it had previously been unknown, first in Guinea and then in Liberia and Sierra Leone. Over the next two years, it

Left: Infographics from the CDC, highlighting how to stop ebola outbreaks; and clarifying how the virus is transmitted.

proceeded to go global, spreading to Mali, Nigeria and Senegal, and then out of Africa to Italy, Spain, the United Kingdom and the United States, where it affected people other than laboratory workers.

In the summer of 2014, panic seized the developed world, with ebola dominating the news agenda for months and being compared with the great plagues of the Middle Ages. From 2014 to 2016, 28,616 people across the world contracted the disease and 11,310 of them died but – despite the terror and the headlines in the Western world – the vast majority of cases were in West Africa, where the long-term effects on the affected societies have been devastating.

In 2016, the World Health Organization (WHO) declared the 2014 pandemic at an end and ebola, for the time being at least, no longer appeared a threat to the West. However, ebola broke out again in a remote part of the DRC in the summer of 2017, infecting eight people, four of whom died. Despite the WHO's announcement, it is a highly debated question as to when a devastating epidemic such as ebola is over as subsequent small outbreaks could be the tail end of an epidemic or a new incidence.

Index cases

How the first person in an outbreak – the index case, or 'patient zero' – catches ebola is still a mystery. While contact with an infected animal such as a fruit bat, monkey or ape, known as the natural reservoir host, has been suggested, no animal has been implicated as a trigger for these outbreaks. A natural reservoir host carries the disease but either doesn't develop it themselves or has only a subclinical infection – in other words, they have no symptoms and suffer no noticeable harm.

In Yambuku, patient zero was thought to be a man who was given an injection for malaria at the mission clinic and later developed symptoms of ebola. Despite an intensive search, no definite link was found between the DRC outbreak and that in Sudan. However, people could and did make the trip between Nzara and the Yambuku area in not more than four days, so it was possible for an infected person to have travelled from Nzara to Yambuku and transferred the virus to a needle at the hospital while receiving an injection at the outpatient clinic.

In the 2014 epidemic, the index case is believed to be a two-year-old boy who died in Guinea in December 2013. He infected his mother, three-year-old sister and grandmother, and the virus then spread to another village among people who had attended the grandmother's funeral. How the boy caught the disease is not known, but an animal bite is thought most likely.

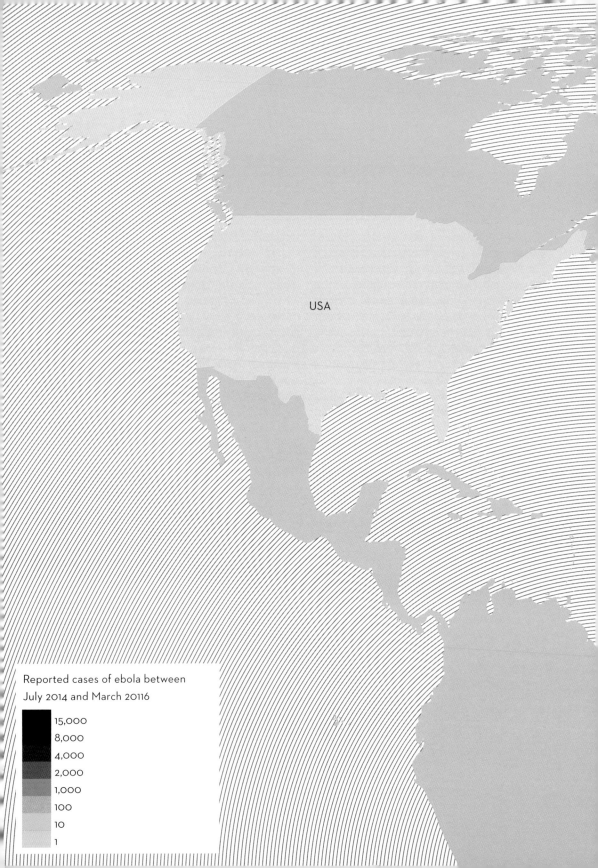

USA

Reported cases of ebola between
July 2014 and March 20116

15,000
8,000
4,000
2,000
1,000
100
10
1

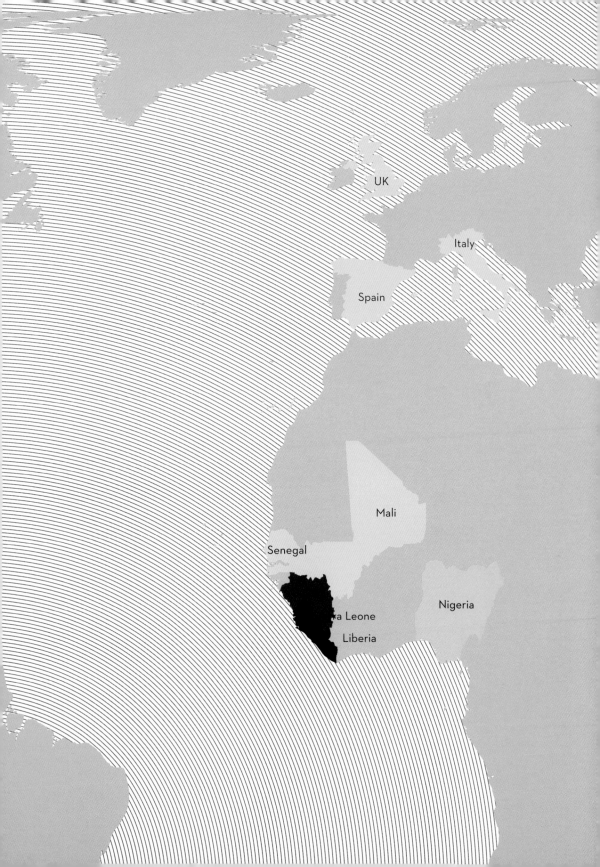

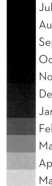

Spread of ebola around the globe
between July 2014 and May 2015

July 2014
August
September
October
November
December
January 2015
February
March
April
May 2015

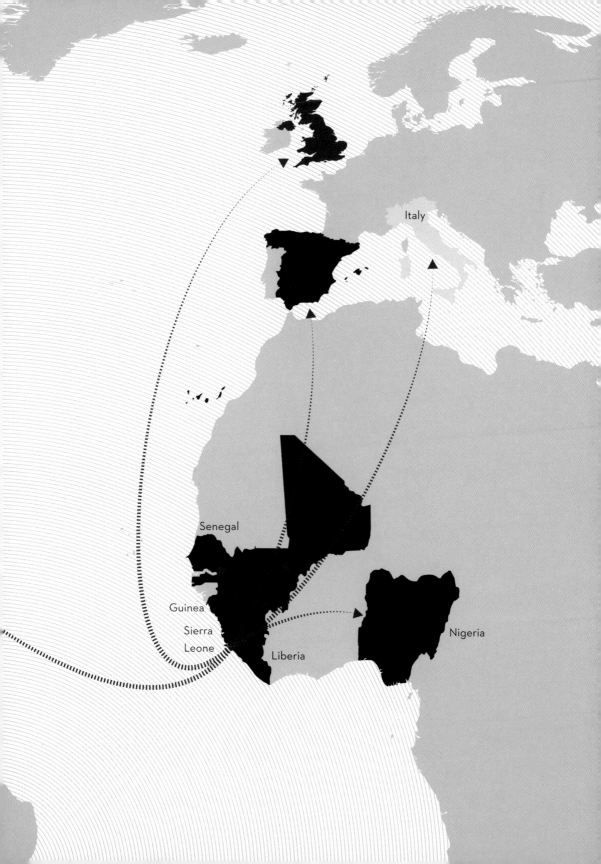

Italy

Senegal

Guinea

Sierra
Leone

Liberia

Nigeria

HIV and AIDS

|||||||||||||||||||

Causal agent	Human immunodeficiency virus (HIV), which exposes the body to a range of conditions, known as acquired immunodeficiency syndrome, or AIDS
Transmission	Anal and vaginal sex and sharing needles and syringes. Less common: mother to child transmission during pregnancy, childbirth or breastfeeding.
Symptoms	Flu-like symptoms. In later stages, symptoms from a range of conditions, including pneumonia.
Deaths	By the end of 2016, HIV and AIDS had killed more than thirty-five million people
Prevalence	Worldwide but the vast majority of cases and deaths are in sub-Saharan Africa
Prevention	Medication (pre-exposure prophylaxis or PrEP) for people at high risk; 'safe sex' practices and needle exchange programmes for intravenous drug users
Treatment	Combination drugs, known as antiretroviral therapy or HAART
Global strategy	Health education to reduce risk-taking behaviours, preventive medication for those at high risk and making anti-retroviral therapy available in the developing world

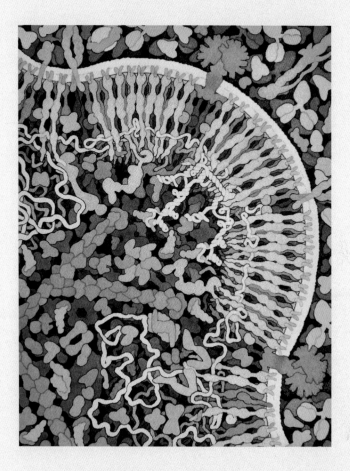

Illustration of HIV during one
of the points in its viral life cycle; here
shows its assembly and budding.

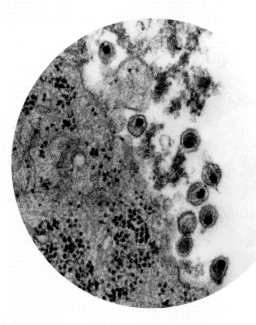

Above: *Microscopic image of HIV.*

In 1999, President Daniel Arap Moi of Kenya spelled out his fears about the epidemic that was engulfing his country. 'AIDS is not just a serious threat to our social and economic development', he said. 'It is a real threat to our very existence.'

HIV and AIDS make up the deadliest epidemic that humankind has ever experienced, according to the United Nations. By the end of 2016, it had devastated countries across sub-Saharan Africa and killed more than thirty-five million people around the globe – including film stars and pop idols but mostly some of the poorest of the poor. This epidemic created terror across continents and brought with it a stigma that would take decades to overcome.

The human immunodeficiency virus, or HIV, is thought to have its origins in West Africa, where the pathogen jumped species from primates to humans in the early twentieth century. By the 1960s, about two thousand people in Africa may have been infected. The earliest known case in a human being was found in a blood sample taken in 1959 from a man in Kinshasa in the Democratic Republic of the Congo. How he became infected, no one knows.

Until the 1980s, when the disease broke out in the United States, it is not known how many people were infected with HIV. By 1980, though, the virus may already have spread to five continents – North America, South America, Europe, Africa and Australia – infecting between one hundred thousand and three hundred thousand people.

First reported US cases

The disease was officially recorded on 5 June 1981. That day, the US Centers for Disease Control and Prevention (CDC) reported that a rare lung infection then called *Pneumocystis carinii* pneumonia (now known as *pneumocystis* pneumonia – PCP), had been diagnosed in five young, previously healthy, gay men in Los Angeles. All of the men were also found to have other unusual infections, which suggested a problem with their immune systems. Two had already died.

The scientists looking for explanations for this strange phenomenon but could find no obvious links between the men. The five didn't know each other. They had no known common contacts and they knew of no sexual partners with similar illnesses. Two said that they had frequent sexual contact with various men. All said they inhaled drugs and one used intravenous drugs.

Within days, doctors across the United States were reporting similar cases, and at the same time reports began coming in of a rare aggressive cancer, Kaposi's sarcoma, in New York and California. Again, all of those affected were gay men. By the end of the year, 270 cases of what was clearly some kind of severe immune deficiency had been reported, 121 of them fatal.

The following year, the CDC coined the term AIDS – acquired immune deficiency syndrome – which it defined as 'a disease at least moderately predictive of a defect in cell-mediated immunity, occurring in a person with no known case for diminished resistance to that disease'.

In fact, by June 1981 roughly 20 per cent of the gay population of San Francisco are believed to have been infected by what

Below: ACT UP activists hang a 'silence = death' banner on the White House gates in 1992.

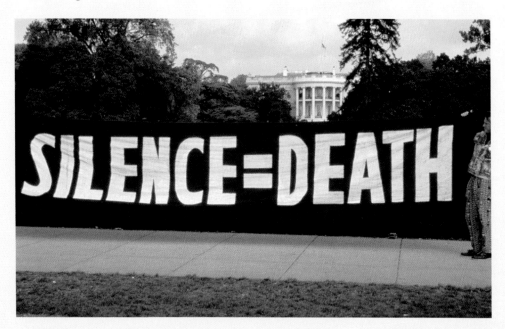

Reported cases of AIDS in the
US between 1981 and 2000

Time period

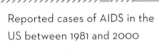

1981–1987

1988–1992

1993–1995

1996–2000

Number of cases

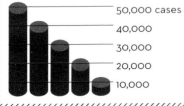

50,000 cases

40,000

30,000

20,000

10,000

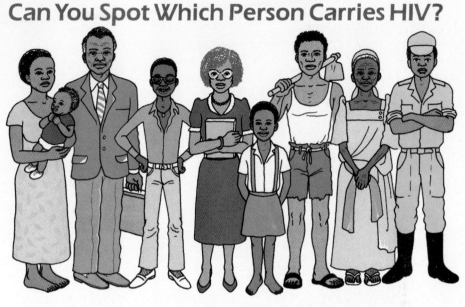

Can You Spot Which Person Carries HIV?

The Answer is NO! The AIDS-Virus can hide in a person's blood for many years. People who carry HIV may look and feel healthy, but they can still pass HIV to others!

Adapted from the Uganda School Health Kit on AIDS Control (Item 5) Ministry of Education, Ministry of Health (AIDS Control Programme), UNICEF Kampala

was later identified as the causative agent. It is also thought that people were already dying of AIDS in New York in the 1970s, mostly homeless and marginalised people.

Cases emerged among other groups such as babies who had received blood transfusions and women whose male partners had AIDS. The data showed, however, that the majority of those affected were homosexual men with multiple sexual partners as well as those who injected drugs, haemophiliacs, and, most strangely, Haitians.

The stigma of AIDS

Haitians living in the United States and people living in Haiti diagnosed with AIDS in 1982 didn't fall into one of the classic

Above: Ugandan poster highlighting the difficulties of spotting who carries the HIV virus, c. 1995.

at-risk groups, so they were singled out as a distinct group of their own. Researchers later discovered that Haitians were no more susceptible to AIDS than anyone else but by then terrible damage had been done to the economy, particularly the tourist industry in that desperately poor country, and the Haitian community in the United States had been the target of much discrimination.

The preponderance of AIDS among homosexual men led to it being dubbed 'the gay plague', echoing old ideas about sexuality and morality, with some people claiming, as with many epidemic diseases

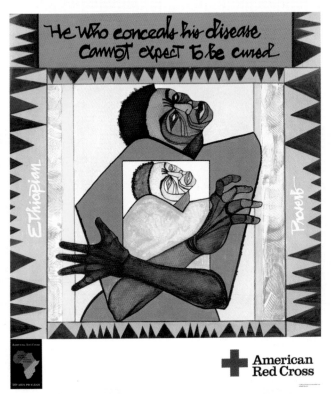

He who conceals his disease cannot expect to be cured

Ethiopian

Proverb

American Red Cross

Left: Poster advertising the American Red Cross HIV/AIDS program, 1992.

in the Middle Ages, that it was God's punishment. This, combined with the mystery about how it was spread, resulted in the diagnosis being seen as shameful and patients regarded as 'untouchable'.

Some people lost their jobs and many were ostracised. Doctors warned that this was deterring those at risk from coming forward to be tested, thus increasing the risk of spread. In 1987, the United States began testing everyone who applied for a visa and those who were found to be positive for the disease were banned from entering the country.

Discovery of the virus

Meanwhile as more evidence emerged, scientists said the culprit was probably an infectious agent, most likely a virus. In September 1983, the CDC announced that AIDS was not spread by casual contact, food, water, air nor by contact with surfaces in the environment. The most likely modes of transmission were sexual contact and blood or blood products. It later transpired that the cells in the rectum are much more susceptible to HIV than those in the vagina, making anal sex eighteen times riskier.

That same year, Luc Montagnier in France isolated a pathogen he named lymphadenopathy-associated virus, later to be known as human immunodeficiency virus or HIV. There was a huge dispute over who then identified HIV as the caused of AIDS, Montagnier and a colleague, or Robert Gallo or Jay Levy in the United

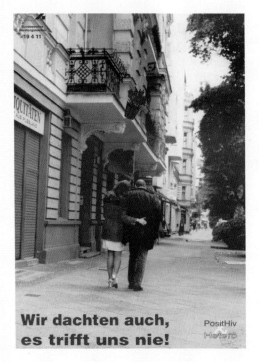

Wir dachten auch, PositHiv
es trifft uns nie!

Above: German poster from the 1990s warning heterosexual people about the dangers of HIV.

States, but in 2008 the two French researchers received the Nobel prize for the discovery.

AIDS is not a single disease but the name given to a group of conditions, such as *Pneumocystis* pneumonia and Karposi's sarcoma, to which people infected with HIV are susceptible because of the specific damage that the virus does to their immune systems. When an individual who is HIV-positive develops one or more of these illnesses, they are given a diagnosis of AIDS.

Celebrities such as film star Rock Hudson, musicians Freddie Mercury and Liberace, ballet dancer Rudolf Nureyev and tennis star Arthur Ashe all died of AIDS-related conditions. In some cases, as with Liberace, the cause of their death was covered up for long after they died. Freddie Mercury announced that he had AIDS only on the day before his death, leading to criticism that he should have used his fame to help break down the taboo about the disease.

African epidemic

While scientists in the West were puzzling over a condition that was largely seen as affecting homosexual men – although in the early days in Europe it was also found among African immigrants with no known risk factors – a heterosexual epidemic broke out in Central Africa, the continent where HIV is believed to have emerged. By 1988 women accounted for half of the adults with HIV in sub-Saharan Africa.

HIV probably reached Eastern Africa – Uganda, Rwanda, Burundi, Tanzania and Kenya – in the 1970s but didn't hit epidemic levels there until the early 1980s. Once established though, it spread fast. Factors such as migration for work, a high ratio of men in the towns and cities and the low status of women, meant that the disease was more devastating there than in West Africa. In Nairobi, 85 per cent of sex workers were infected with HIV in 1986.

Uganda was hit particularly hard. The first warning was a surge in a severe wasting condition known locally as 'slim disease', as well as opportunistic infections including Kaposi's sarcoma. By then doctors knew about the AIDS cases in the United States. 'But we just could not connect a disease in white, homosexual males in San Francisco to the thing that we were staring at', said David Serwadda of the Uganda Cancer Institute.

The epidemic moved south, and by the end of the decade Malawi, Zambia,

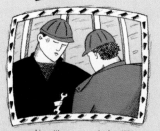

You **cannot** catch the HIV virus by:

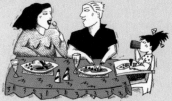

working with someone who has HIV

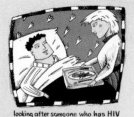

living with someone who has HIV

looking after someone who has HIV

Zimbabwe and Botswana were on the verge of overtaking East Africa as the focus of the epidemic. By 2001, President Festus Mogae of Botswana spelled out the same desperate message as his counterpart in Kenya two years earlier. 'We are threatened with extinction', he said. 'People are dying in chillingly high numbers. It is a crisis of the first magnitude.'

Initially, the World Health Organization (WHO) was slow to respond, as indeed it would be in the ebola crisis of 2014–16. In 1985, the WHO's director general, Halfdan Mahler, told African countries not to make

the disease a priority. 'AIDS is not spreading like bush fire in Africa', he said. 'It is malaria and other tropical diseases that are killing millions of children every day.' The following year, however, Mahler apologised and put a global action plan in place. 'We're running scared', he said. 'We stand naked in front of a very serious pandemic, as mortal as any pandemic there ever has been.'

The response from African countries themselves was patchy. Some were reluctant to admit to an epidemic for fear of creating panic or discouraging tourism, as had happened in Haiti. In the Congo, the press was initially banned from mentioning the subject and in Zimbabwe doctors were ordered not to write AIDS on death certificates, although Zimbabwe was the first developing country to begin blood screening. And health educators met resistance in promoting the safe sex message. Some religious leaders were reluctant to endorse condoms, for example.

Medication for HIV and AIDS

In 1985, the US government and the WHO hosted the first International AIDS conference, and in 1988, 1 December was designated World AIDS Day. The 1990s brought huge steps forward in dealing with HIV/AIDS. In 1996, a highly effective combination therapy known as highly active anti-retroviral therapy (HAART) became available in rich countries. Death rates there dropped by 84 per cent over the next four years, which led scientists to predict that HIV/AIDS would soon become a chronic, manageable condition like diabetes.

However, most people with HIV lived in Africa where the drugs weren't affordable, although controversially many of those drugs were tested on African populations. In 1999, after a sustained campaign, the pharmaceutical companies agreed to allow poorer countries either to produce the drugs themselves or to import them at lower cost. Not every country had the facilities to produce drugs, however, or the ability to manage large-scale treatment programmes or was able to afford even the cheaper drugs.

Delivering medicines to remote parts of Africa also proved a stumbling block although Joep Lange, president of the International AIDS Society, made the point: 'If we can get cold Coca Cola and beer to every remote corner of Africa, it should not be impossible to do the same with drugs.'

In 2012, the WHO issued guidelines for prescribing a preventive medication, pre-exposure prophylaxis (PrEP), to healthy people who are at high risk of HIV. Highly effective when taken regularly, it has been greeted by some as marking the beginning of the end of the disease. However, its use is controversial in Europe and North America. In the UK, for example, there is a debate about whether the cash-strapped NHS should fund the therapy, with opponents arguing that those at high risk should take responsibility and change their behaviours.

In 2017, scientists announced that a child born with HIV and given a short course of treatment had remained healthy for nine years without further drugs, giving hope to other children born with the virus. By then, around 40 million people had HIV, 2.1 million of them children. Most of those children lived in sub-Saharan Africa and had been infected by their mothers during pregnancy, childbirth or breastfeeding.

Reported number of people
living with HIV in 2016

19,400,000
6,100,000
5,100,000
2,110,000
2,100,000
1,600,000
230,000

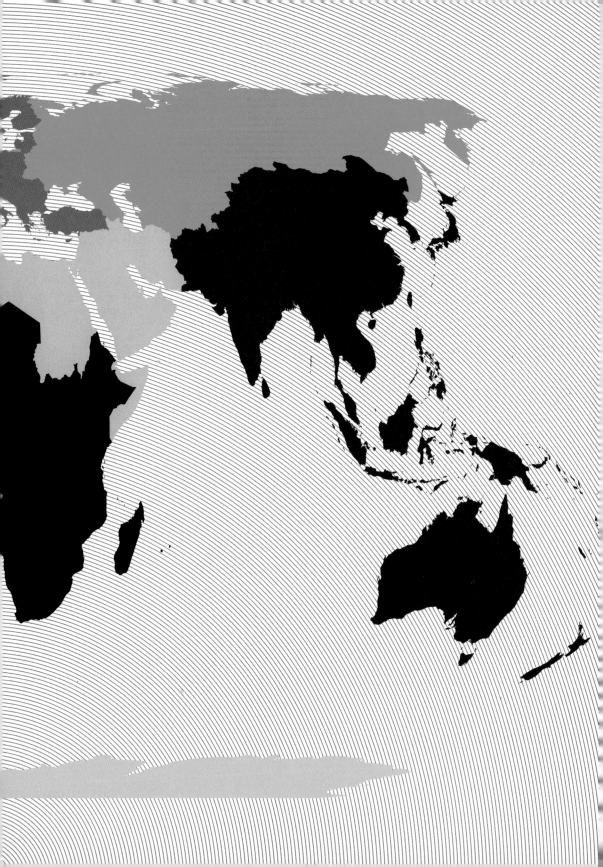

Syphilis

||||||||||||||||||

Causal agent	Bacterium *Treponema pallidum*
Transmission	Person to person through sexual contact
Symptoms	A sore followed by skin rash and inflammation of the mucous membranes and lymph glands. A few cases eventually progress to tertiary syphilis, which attacks bones, tissues, the central nervous system, the cardiovascular system and the brain.
Prevalence	Worldwide. Was close to eradication in the US but is now on the rise again.
Prevention	'Safe sex' practices
Treatment	Antibiotics
Global strategy	Health education, regular screening of those at high risk and fast treatment

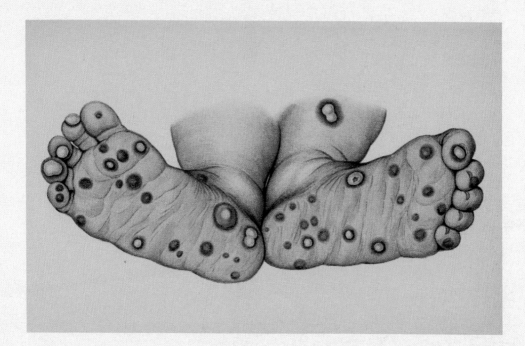

Illustration of congenital syphilis,
affecting a baby's feet, 1898.

No sooner had syphilis struck Europe at the end of the fifteenth century than a blame game was underway. The French named it the Neapolitan or the Spanish disease; the English, Italians and Germans called it the French disease; the Russians, the Polish disease; the Poles and the Persians, the Turkish disease. And the Turks took discrimination beyond nationality, dubbing it the Christian disease.

As the infection continued to spread fast around the world, the Tahitians would blame the British; the Indians, the Portuguese; and the Japanese would hold the Chinese responsible.

Unknown beginnings

Experts have long argued about where syphilis first emerged. Many assumed it had its origins in the Americas, as little trace of the infection had been found elsewhere before Christopher Columbus's arrival in 1492. His men were thought to have then brought it back with them into Europe. In 2000, however, the skeletal remains of monks dating back to the fourteenth century, buried at a priory in Hull, were found to show signs of the disease. The fact that so many skeletons were affected led the researchers to conclude that the disease was widely present in England at that time, but this is still under debate.

Some ancient sculptures in the Americas are thought to depict syphilis victims, and some pre-Columbian human remains have bone lesions that might indicate the disease. The Spaniards claimed that when they arrived, Native Americans described to them what was a familiar disease that sounded like syphilis and said that the local population seemed to have some immunity.

Early written accounts

Also known simply as the pox, syphilis takes its modern name from a sixteenth-century poem by an Italian physician. Girolamo Fracastoro tells the tale of a shepherd boy, Syphilus, who insulted the Greek god Apollo and was punished with a horrible disease: 'He first wore buboes dreadful to the sight. First felt strange pains and sleepless passed the night.'

The first reports of syphilis came in 1495 when the French invaded the Kingdom of Naples. The fifty thousand-strong army, mostly mercenaries from across Europe, was suddenly struck down with a previously unknown and terrible sickness. It was an acute condition that attacked fast and laid its victims low, unlike the slow-developing infection known today.

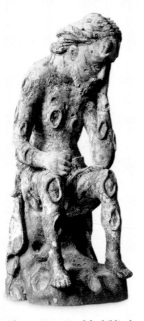

Above: Statuette of the biblical character Job, showing syphilis ulcers.

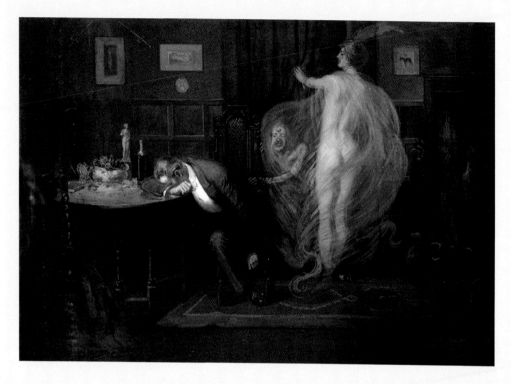

When the Neapolitans counter-at-tacked, many of the invaders were too ill to fight and were forced into retreat. The mercenaries returned home to their various countries, taking with them the new disease. 'On their flippant way through Italy, the French carelessly picked up Genoa, Naples and syphilis,' quipped the French writer Voltaire. 'Then they were thrown out and deprived of Naples and Genoa. But they did not lose everything – syphilis went with them.'

By the end of the year, an epidemic had spread throughout France, Switzerland and Germany. The Holy Roman Emperor pronounced it a punishment from God, a charge that would be laid against syphilis for centuries. The disease meanwhile travelled on at speed, first to England and Scotland and then to Scandinavia,

Above: Syphilis *by Richard Tennant Cooper, 1912.*

Hungary, Greece, Poland and Russia. By 1520 explorers had taken it across the world to India, Africa, the Middle East, China, Japan and Oceania.

At that time, syphilis killed faster, spread more easily and carried a higher mortality rate, perhaps because the strain was more virulent. The Dutch theologian Erasmus said it was by far the most destructive of all diseases, asking 'What contagion does thus invade the whole body, so much resist medical art ... and so cruelly tortures the patient?'

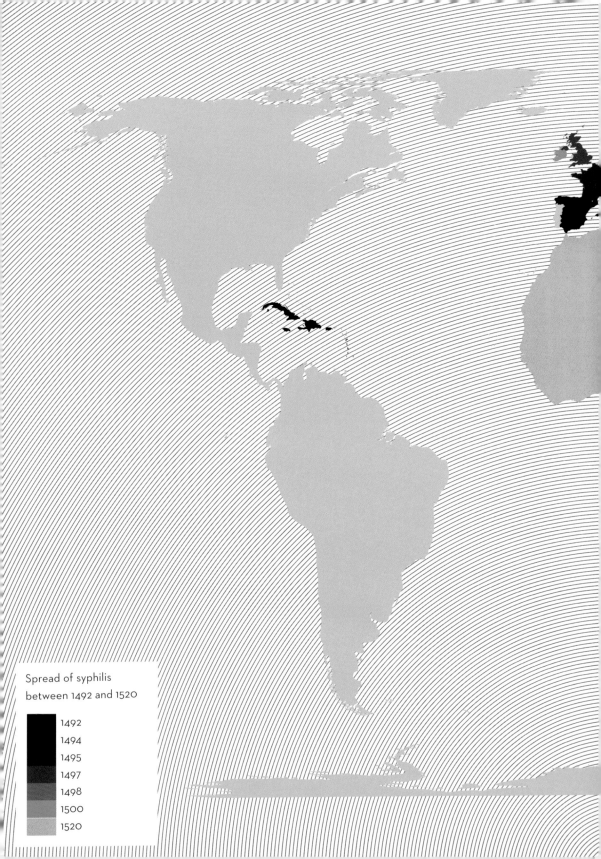

Spread of syphilis
between 1492 and 1520

1492
1494
1495
1497
1498
1500
1520

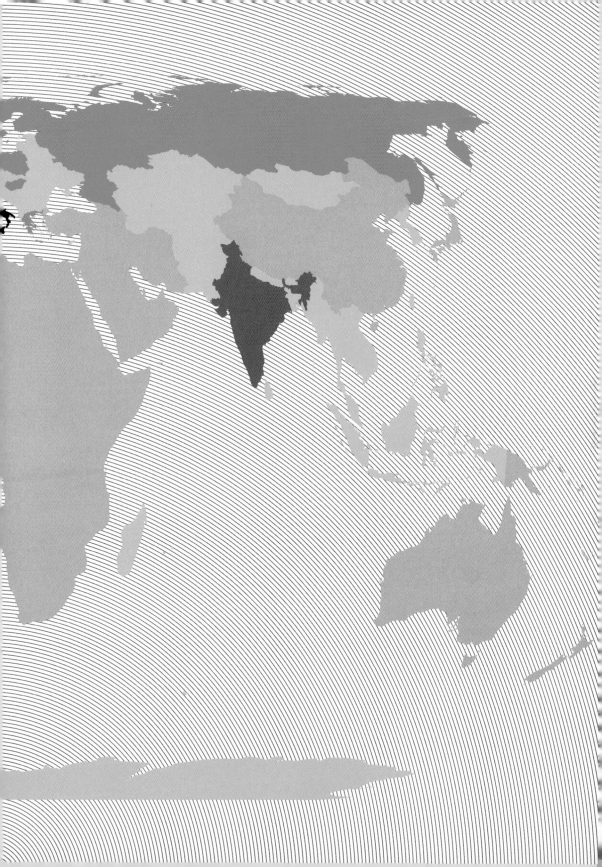

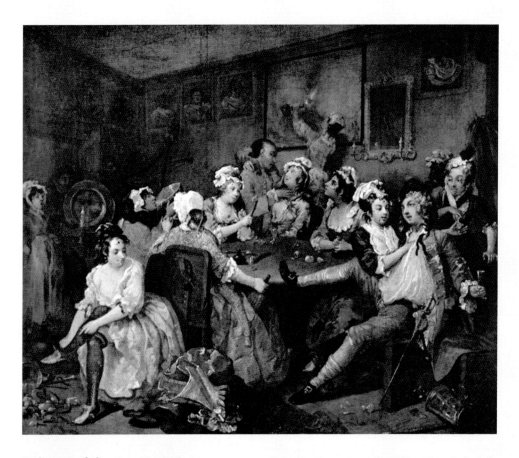

'A disease of the promiscuous'

Syphilis is spread mainly through sexual contact when the bacterium *Treponema pallidum* is transferred into broken skin or mucous membranes during intercourse. The condition known as congenital syphilis is found in newborn babies who have been infected by their mother in the womb. Unlike many contagious diseases, whose transmission remained a mystery for centuries, doctors realised fairly quickly how syphilis was passed on. Stopping it, however, was another matter.

In fifteenth-century Europe, governments reacted by trying to clamp down on what was seen as promiscuity and, in

Above The Tavern Scene *by William Hogarth, from the series 'A Rake's Progress'. The black spots on the women may suggest they have syphilis.*

particular, on prostitution. In 1546, King Henry VIII attempted to close the notorious Southwark 'stews', or brothels, on the south bank of the Thames. Ironically, the idea later took root that the ageing king's suppurating leg ulcer and increasing mental instability were due to tertiary – or third-stage – syphilis, but this has now been discounted. By the eighteenth century, references to the use of the 'condum' as a form of protection began to crop up.

From the early sixteenth to the early twentieth centuries, the main treatment for syphilis was mercury, sometimes taken in liquid form but more usually applied to the skin ulcers in an ointment. Patients were sometimes placed next to a hot fire, rubbed with the ointment and left to sweat. The procedure was repeated several times a day for a month or more. Doctors also used guaiacum resin, an extract from a tropical plant. Guaiacum didn't work but mercury did help to some extent with the skin problems. The side effects, however, could be terrible, and patients sometimes died from mercury poisoning. Treatment often went on for years, leading to the saying, 'A night with Venus and a lifetime with Mercury'.

William Hogarth's series of engravings 'A Harlot's Progress', completed in 1732, trace the downfall of a country curate's daughter who comes to London and falls into prostitution. In the final scene, Moll lies dying either from syphilis or from the effects of treatment, her teeth on a piece of paper, having fallen out because of the mercury.

Opinion was divided over whether syphilis was a divine punishment. Some people thought that sufferers should be dealt with harshly and even refused medical treatment, but not everyone agreed. The seventeenth-century English physician Thomas Sydenham argued that patients' morals were not a matter for doctors. It was the physician's duty to treat everyone, he said. However, in nineteenth-century Britain most hospitals refused to take syphilis cases. They went instead to the workhouse infirmaries, where they were isolated in what were known as 'foul' or 'lock' wards. The Lock Hospital opened in 1747 near Hyde Park Corner to treat syphilis and gonorrhoea, the first specialist voluntary hospital in London and the first of a chain of clinics in Britain and the empire. By the mid-nineteenth century, most of the larger army bases in India had a Lock hospital.

In the 1860s, Britain brought in the Contagious Diseases Acts that allowed a woman identified by the police as a 'common prostitute' to be forced to undergo regular internal examination. If she was found to have syphilis or gonorrhoea, she would be placed in a Lock hospital for up to nine months. In certain military towns, any woman could be forcibly inspected. Men were not examined, however, because the authorities deemed they wouldn't accept it. The laws were controversial from the start and were repealed in 1886.

Fluctuations in more recent times

By the early eighteenth century, and perhaps before, syphilis had changed from the virulent epidemic disease that had devastated the French army in Naples to resemble the condition of today, although some of the cases recorded as syphilis might, in fact, have been other, milder sexually transmitted diseases. Not until the nineteenth century was it established beyond doubt that syphilis and gonorrhoea were separate diseases, not different forms of the same illness.

From the mid-nineteenth to the mid-twentieth centuries the incidence also declined in industrialised countries, except in wartime. During the two world wars and the Korean and Vietnam wars, cases of syphilis and other sexually transmitted diseases (STDs) rose sharply. In the US army, STDs were the second most common reason for disability and absence from

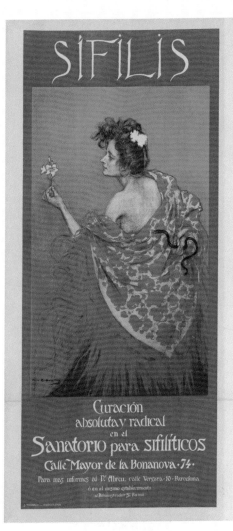

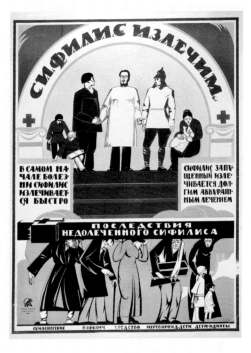

Above: An advertisement for Dr Abreu's sanatorium for syphilitics in Barcelona, c. 1900.

Above right: USSR poster, c. 1920s. The top depicts how syphilis can be easily treated in its early stages; the bottom shows the consequences of leaving it untreated.

Opposite: Turkish poster depicting the symptoms, transmission and consequences of syphilis.

duty in the First World War, surpassed only by the Spanish flu epidemic of 1918–19. When the hostilities stopped, the incidence dropped. After the Second World War, syphilis was one of the main drivers for the production of the new antibiotic penicillin, particularly in Europe.

In 2018, syphilis was still causing concern. The previous year the US Centers for Disease Control and Prevention (CDC) reported that it was on the rise again in the United States after being close to elimination. This increase has been found to correlate with a change in the sex education message to one of promoting abstinence, where advice about protection is deemed unnecessary. Men accounted for more than 89 per cent of all cases of first-stage (primary) and second-stage (secondary) syphilis cases in 2016 in the United States, mostly in men who had sex with men.

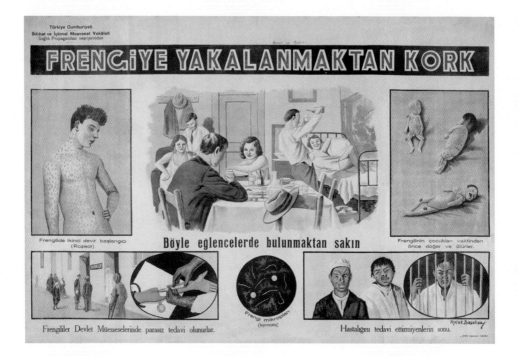

FRENGİYE YAKALANMAKTAN KORK

Frengilide ikinci devir başlangıcı
(Rozeol)

Böyle eğlencelerde bulunmaktan sakın

Frengilinin çocukları vaktinden
önce doğar ve ölürler.

Frengililer Devlet Müesseselerinde parasız tedavi olunurlar.

Frengi mikropları
(Ispiroceta)

Hastalığını tedavi ettirmiyenlerin sonu.

There has also been a 'troubling rise' in congenital syphilis, according to the CDC, although the disease is preventable through routine screening of pregnant women and fast treatment. Rates were eight times higher among infants born to black mothers and 3.9 times higher in infants born to Hispanic mothers compared with infants born to white mothers. Race and Hispanic ethnicity in the United States are linked with factors that affect people's health, including poverty, unemployment and poor education. Those who can't afford basic necessities might have trouble accessing and affording good-quality sexual health services, the CDC reported.

Meanwhile, in England in 2016, rates were at their highest since 1949 and almost double those in 2012. As in the United States, the cases were mainly among men who had sex with men.

In early 2018, two minority and low socio-economic groups in Australia were affected. A child died of congenital syphilis in Queensland, the sixth such death out of thirteen infants born with the infection since 2011. Infectious syphilis was spreading through the country's indigenous communities – the Aboriginal and Torres Strait Islander populations – from Queensland into the Northern Territory, Western Australia and South Australia, and congenital syphilis was also on the rise.

Index

Page numbers in *italics* indicate maps.

Credits

7 'A map taken from a report by Dr. John Snow', Wellcome Collection, CC BY; 13 Wikimedia Commons, URL: https://commons.wikimedia.org/wiki/File:El_Lazarillo_de_Tormes_de_Goya.jpg; 14 Melba Photo Agency/Alamy Stock Photo; 15 'Symptoms of diptheria, in Koplik', Wellcome Collection, CC BY; 19 Mary Evans/Library of Congress; 23 'Charles Kean, ill with flu. Coloured etching', Wellcome Collection, CC BY; 24 'Drawing of the 1918 Influenza: Lymph sinus' by John George Adami, Wellcome Collection, CC BY; 28 'A monster representing an influenza virus hitting a man over the head as he sits in his armchair', pen and ink drawing by Ernest Noble, c. 1918, Wellcome Collection, CC BY; 33 '28 year old woman with leprosy, from the title "Om spedalskhed ... Atlas/udgivet efter foranstaltning of den Kongelige Norske Regjerings Department for det Indre. Tegningerne udförte af J.L. Losting", Authors: Danielssen, D. C. (Daniel Cornelius), 1815–94 and Losting, Johan Ludvig, 1810–76 and Boeck, W. (Wilhelm), 1808–75', Wellcome Collection, CC BY; 34 'The Leprosy Man' woodcut, akg-images; 35 'Leprosy of the skin: an Indian man with red patches on his chest. Watercolour (by Jane Jackson), 1921/1950, after a (painting) by Ernest Muir, c. 1921', Wellcome Collection, CC BY; 39 'Leprosy poster, India, 1950s' by Hind Kusht Nivaran Sangh, Wellcome Collection, CC BY; 43 VintageMedStock/Alamy Stock Photo; 44 Scott Camazine/Alamy Stock Photo; 45 Chronicle/Alamy Stock Photo; 46 CCI Archives/Science Photo Library; 47 Australian War Memorial/Wikimedia Commons, URL: https://commons.wikimedia.org/wiki/File:HMS_Dido_(1869)_AWM_302178.jpeg; 49 'Four children, two with measles, in the same bed: their mother tells the district nurse that there is no risk of infection', wood engraving by Starr Wood, 1915, Wellcome Collection, CC BY; 53 VintageMedStock/Alamy Stock Photo; 54 Gado Images/Alamy Stock Photo; 55 © Florilegius/Getty Images; 58 'A country vicar visiting a family where a child has been suffering from scarlet fever', wood engraving by Claude Alin Shepperson, Wellcome Collection, CC BY; 61 Scott Camazine/Alamy Stock Photo; 62 Phanie/Alamy Stock Photo; 68 Luis Enrique Ascui/Stringer/Getty Images; 69 Iain Masterton/Alamy Stock Photo; 71 'Edward Jenner vaccinating patients against smallpox' by James Gillray, Wellcome Collection, CC BY; 73 'Smallpox, textured illustration, Japanese manuscript, c. 1720', Wellcome Collection, CC BY; 74 'Ships used as smallpox isolation hospitals', Wellcome Collection, CC BY; 75 'Gloucester smallpox epidemic, 1896: a ward in the isolation hospital', photograph by H.C.F., 1896, Wellcome Collection, CC BY; 77 'St Pancras Smallpox Hospital, London: housed in a tented camp at Finchley', watercolour by Frank Collins, 1881, Wellcome Collection, CC BY; 81 'A health visitor holding a small child, promoting a campaign against tuberculosis and infant mortality', colour process print by Jules Marie Auguste Leroux, Wellcome Collection, CC BY; 82 Hulton Archive/Stringer/Getty Images; 89 'Liverpool's x-ray campaign against tuberculosis', lithograph, c. 1960, Wellcome Collection, CC BY; 93 'John Bull defending Britain against the invasion of cholera; satirizing resistance to the Reform Bill', coloured lithograph, c. 1832, Wellcome Collection, CC BY; 94 'A cholera patient experimenting with remedies', coloured etching by Robert Cruikshank, c. 1832, Wellcome Collection, CC BY; 95 'Actual & supposed routes of Cholera from Hindoostan to Europe', Wellcome Collection, CC BY; 97 'John Snow, 1856', Wellcome Collection, CC BY; 98 'A map taken from a report by Dr. John Snow', Wellcome Collection, CC BY; 103 'Soldier suffering from dysentery',Wellcome Collection, CC BY; 106 Universal History Archive/Getty Images; 109 'Man suffering from typhoid', Wellcome Collection, CC BY; 110 Shutterstock; 111 'The angel of death (a winged skeletal creature) drops some deadly substances into a river near a town; representing typhoid', watercolour, 1912, by Richard Tennant Cooper, Wellcome Collection, CC BY; 112 Science & Society Picture Library/Getty Images; 113 Mary Evans Picture Library; 117 'Anti-typhoid vaccination in World War I', photograph, Wellcome Collection, CC BY; 121 'Lady suffering from malaria', Abb 7, page 82, Wellcome Collection, CC BY; 122 'Illustrations of parasites that cause malaria, 1901', by Giovanni Battista Grassi, Wellcome Collection, CC BY; 124 'Map of the world, showing positions of malaria', Wellcome Collection, CC BY; 125 'The malaria mosquito forming the eye-sockets of a skull, rep', by Abram Games, Wellcome Collection, CC BY; 126 'World Health Organisation Interim Committee on malaria', photograph, 1947, Wellcome Collection, CC BY; 133 'A physician wearing a seventeenth-century plague preventive costume', watercolour, Wellcome Collection, CC BY; 134 'The dance of death', lithograph after A. Dauzats, 1831, Wellcome Collection, CC BY; 135 Wikimedia Commons, URL: https://commons.wikimedia.org/wiki/File:Pieter_Bruegel_the_Elder_-_The_Triumph_of_Death_-_WGA3389.jpg; 139 'A cart for transporting the dead in London during the great', by George Cruikshank, Wellcome Collection, CC BY; 143 'Soldiers suffering from typhus, lying in the streets', lithograph by E. Leroux after A. Raffet, by Denis-Auguste-Marie Raffet, Wellcome Collection, CC BY; 144 Mary Evans Picture Library; 147 'After the defeat of the White Army, a new white peril threatens in the form of the typhus louse, against which the Red soldiers fight by washing themselves and their clothes vigorously', colour lithograph, c. 1921, Wellcome Collection, CC BY; 151 'Different stages of yellow fever, 1820', Wellcome Collection, CC BY; 152 'Yellow fever: section of the liver of a patient infected with yellow fever', watercolour, c. 1920, Wellcome Collection, CC BY; 153 'A parodic cosmological diagram

showing opposing aspects of the life of colonialists in Jamaica – langorous noons and the hells of yellow fever', coloured aquatint by A.J., 1800, Wellcome Collection, CC BY; 154 Mary Evans Picture Library/Everett Collection; 155 'A yellow quarantine flag, signalling yellow fever, raised on a ship anchored at sea some distance from a port', watercolour by E. Schwarz, c. 1920/1950, Wellcome Collection, CC BY; 161 'Zika virus, illustration' by RCSB Protein Data Bank, Wellcome Collection, CC BY; 162 Cultura Creative (RF)/Alamy Stock Photo; 167 Konstantin Nechaev/ Alamy Stock Photo; 173; 'R.W.Lovett, Treatment of Infantile Paralysis', Wellcome Collection, CC BY; 175 Wikimedia Commons, URL: https://commons.wikimedia.org/wiki/File:Roosevelt_in_a_wheelchair.jpg; 177 left 'Poster issued by the British Ministry of Health for the vaccination against Polio', colour lithograph, c 1940, Wellcome Collection, CC BY; 177 right 'CDC Symbol of Public Health, Wellbe', 1963, Science History Images/ Alamy Stock Photo; 178 Fox Photos/Stringer/Getty Images; 179 World History Archive/Alamy Stock Photo;
183 'Cross section through an ebola virus particle, illustration', by David S. Goodsell, RCSB Protein Data Bank, Wellcome Collection, CC BY; 184 Cultura RM/Alamy Stock Photo; 185 'The Ebola virus' by Odra Noel, Wellcome Collection, CC BY-NC; 188 Centers for Disease Control and Prevention; 195 'HIV assembly and budding, HIV viral life cycle', illustration by David S. Goodsell, The Scripps Research Institute, Wellcome Collection, CC BY; 196 Scott Camazine/Alamy Stock Photo; 197 Jeffrey Markowitz/Getty Images; 199 'The difficulty in spotting who carries the HIV virus', poster by UNICEF Uganda, Uganda Ministry of Education and Uganda Ministry of Health, Wellcome Collection, CC BY-NC; 200 'American Red Cross HIV/ AIDS program', American Red Cross, Wellcome Collection, CC BY-NC; 201 'Warning about the dangers of HIV and heterosexual people', colour lithograph by Positiv & Hetero, Wellcome Collection, CC BY-NC; 202 'Ways in which you cannot catch the HIV virus from working, living or looking after someone who has HIV', one of a series of fact sheets about AIDS and HIV, colour lithograph, c.1990–99, Wellcome Collection. CC BY-NC; 207 'Tab 59, Heridary syphilis, baby's feet', from Atlas of syphilis and the veneral diseases by Prof. Dr. Franz Mra ek, Wellcome Collection, CC BY; 208 'Front of Job statue, showing syphilis ulcers', Wellcome Collection, CC BY; 209 'Syphilis', gouache by Richard Tennant Cooper, 1912, Wellcome Collection, CC BY; 212 Wikimedia Commons, URL: https://commons.wikimedia.org/wiki/File:William_Hogarth_027.jpg; 214 left 'A woman representing syphilis; advertising Dr Abreu's sanatorium for syphilitics in Barcelona', colour lithograph by R. Casas, Wellcome Collection, CC BY; 214 right 'Syphilis: the benefits of its medical treatment, contrasted', Wellcome Collection, CC BY; 215 'Syphilis: its symptoms, transmission and consequences in Turkey', colour lithograph by Refet Basokçu, Sihhat ve ' Içtimai Muavenet Vekâleti, Wellcome Collection, CC BY.

While every effort has been made to credit contributors, White Lion Publishing would like to apologise should there have been any omissions or errors, and would be pleased to make the appropriate corrections to future editions of the book.

Map sources

All maps created by Lovell Johns Ltd. Data has been referenced from the following sources: 16–17 *The Strangling Angel: Diphtheria in Hamilton*, ed. D. Ann Herring, Department of Anthropology, McMaster University, Ontario, Canada; 20–21 World Health Organization data, http://www.who.int/immunization/monitoring_surveillance/data/en/; 26–27, 30–31 World Health Organization data, http://www.who.int/influenza/en/, *Textbook of Influenza*, ed. K.G. Nicholson, A.J. Hay, R.B. Webster, Blackwell Science, *World Atlas of Epidemic Diseases*, A. Cliff, P. Haggett, M. Smallman-Raynor, Taylor & Francis Group; 36–37 'Leprosy: Infectious Disease' by Susannah C. J. Kearns and June E. Nash, Britannica.com; 40–41 World Health Organization data, http://apps.who.int/iris/bitstream/handle/10665/258841/WER9235.pdf; 48 *World Atlas of Epidemic Diseases*, A. Cliff, P. Haggett, M. Smallman-Raynor, Taylor & Francis Group; 50 Centers for Disease Control data, Statista; 56–57 World Health Organization data, http://apps.who.int/iris/handle/10665/237884; 64–65, 66–67 World Health Organization data, http://www.who.int/csr/sars/country/2003_08_15/en/; 76 World Health Organization data, http://apps.who.int/iris/bitstream/handle/10665/219809/WER4915.PDF; 78–79 *Smallpox and its Eradication*, F. Fenner, D.A. Henderson, I. Arita, Z. Jezek, I.D. Ladnyi, World Health Organization, 1998; 84–85, 86–87 World Health Organization data, Statista; 96 *On the Mode of Communication of Cholera*, John Snow, M.D., Wellcome Library; 100 World Health Organization data, Statista, Centers for Disease Control; 107 Report on Dysentery in Japan 1897 from US Consul archives; 114–155 'Typhoid fever and paratyphoid fever: Systematic review to estimate global morbidity and mortality for 2010', Geoffrey C. Buckle, Christa L. Fischer Walker, and Robert E. Black, © 2012 by the Journal of Global Health; 128–129, 130–131 World Health Organization data, Statista; 136–137 'Black Death', Encyclopedia Britannica, *World Atlas of Epidemic Diseases*, A. Cliff, P. Haggett, M. Smallman-Raynor, Taylor & Francis Group; 140 World Health Organization data, http://apps.who.int/iris/bitstream/handle/10665/259556/Ex-PlagueMadagascar04122017.pdf; 148–149 World Health Organization data, http://apps.who.int/iris/handle/10665/237185; 156–157 Centers for Disease Control data, Statista; 159 World Health Organization data, http://www.afro.who.int/sites/default/files/2017-06/angola_yf_sitrep_6june.2016.pdf; 164–165, 168–169 World Health Organization data, http://www.who.int/emergencies/zika-virus/situation-report/6-october-2016/en/; 174 Statistics from the Official Reports of the Bureaus of the Department of Health of New York City, 1917; 180–181 World Health Organization data, Global Polio Eradication Initiative, 2017; 186, 190–191, 192–193 World Health Organization data, Statista; 198 Centers for Disease Control data, https://www.cdc.gov/mmwr/preview/mmwrhtml/mm5021a2.htm; 204–205 UNAIDS data, Statista; 210–211 'Syphilis – its early history and treatment until Penicillin and the debate on its origins', John Frith, *Journal of Military and Veteran's Health*, Volume 20, no. 4, November 2012.